Psychopathology

International Journal of Descriptive Psychopathology, Phenomenology and Clinical Diagnostics

Founded 1897 as 'Monatsschrift für Psychiatrie und Neurologie',
continued 1957–1967 as 'Psychiatria et Neurologia'
Founders: C. Wernicke and Th. Ziehen
Successors: K. Bonhoeffer (1912–1938), J. Klaesi (1939–1967), E. Grünthal (1953–1973), N. Petrilowitsch (1968–1970), Th. Spoerri (1971–1973)
continued 1968–1983 as 'Psychiatria Clinica'

Publication data: 'Psychopathology' is published 6 times annually. Volume 24 with 6 issues appears in 1991.

Subscription rates: Subscriptions run for a full calendar year. Prices are given per volume, surface postage included.

Personal subscription: SFr. 238.–, US$ 190.40. (Must be in the name of, billed to, and paid by an individual. Order must be marked 'personal subscription'.)

Institutional subscription: SFr. 340.–, US$ 272.00. (Regular rate.)

Members of various related societies: SFr. 204.– , US$ 163.20.

Airmail postage: SFr. 35.–, US$ 25.00. (Extra per volume.)

Microform subscription: SFr. 170.–. US$ 136.00. (Available exclusively to subscribers of the paper edition.)

Single issues and back volumes: Information on availability and prices can be obtained through the Publisher.

Subscription orders: Orders can be placed at agencies, bookstores, directly with the Publisher S. Karger AG, P.O. Box, CH – 4009 Basel (Switzerland) or with any of the following distributors:

Deutschland, Österreich, Ost-Europa: S. Karger GmbH, Postfach 1724, D – 8034 Germering/München

France: Librairie Luginbühl, 36, bd de Latour-Maubourg, F – 75007 Paris

Great Britain, Ireland: S. Karger Publishers, 1 Torberry Drive, Petersfield, Hampshire GU 31 4HW

USA: S. Karger Publishers, Inc., 26 West Avon Road, P.O. Box 529, Farmington, CT 06085

India, Bangladesh, Sri Lanka: S. Karger India Subscription Agency, B – 5/132 Safdarjung Enclave, New Delhi-110029

Japan: Katakura Libri, Inc., 36-9 Hongo 3-chome, Bunkyo-ku, Tokyo 113

Change of address: Both old and new address should be stated and sent to the subscription source.

Bibliographic indices: This journal is regularly listed in bibliographic services, including *Current Contents*® .

Advertising: Correspondence and rate requests should be addressed to the Publisher.

KARGER

Psychopathology
Printed in Switzerland

S. Karger AG,
Postfach, CH – 4009 Basel (Schweiz)

Erscheint zweimonatlich
pro Jahr 1 Band zu 6 Heften

Submission: Only original papers written in English are considered and should be sent to:

Prof. Dr. P. Berner
Direktor der Psychiatrischen Universitätsklinik
Lazarettgasse 14
A–1090 Wien (Austria)

Manuscripts should be submitted in duplicate (with two sets of illustrations of which one is an original), typewritten double-spaced on one side of the paper, with a wide margin.

Conditions: All manuscripts are subject to editorial review. Manuscripts are received with the explicit understanding that they are not under simultaneous consideration by any other publication. Submission of an article for publication implies the transfer of the copyright from the author to the publisher upon acceptance. Accepted papers become the permanent property of 'Psychopathology' and may not be reproduced by any means, in whole or in part, without the written consent of the publisher. It is the author's responsibility to obtain permission to reproduce illustrations, tables, etc. from other publications.

Arrangement:

Title page: The first page of each paper should indicate the title (main title underlined), the authors' names, and the institute where the work was conducted. A translation of the full title into English and a short title for use as running head are also required.

Abstract: Each paper needs an abstract of up to 10 lines.

Methods: The reader should be able to follow the methods by which the results were obtained, but there is no need of detailed descriptions unless of a genuine innovation.

Results: The results should be described precisely and must be separated from discussion.

Discussion: The discussion should be confined to the interpretation of the results and should not consist of a repetition of them.

Small type: Paragraphs which can or must be set in smaller type (case histories, test methods, etc.) should be indicated with a 'p' (petit) in the margin on the left-hand side.

Footnotes: Avoid footnotes. When essential, they are numbered consecutively and typed at the foot of the appropriate page.

Tables and illustrations: Tables and illustrations (both numbered in Arabic numerals) should be prepared on separate sheets. Tables require a heading and figures a legend, also prepared on a separate sheet. For the reproduction of illustrations, only good drawings and original photographs can be accepted; negatives or photocopies cannot be used. When possible, group several illustrations on one block for reproduction (max. size 140 × 188 mm) or provide crop marks. On the back of each illustration, indicate its number, the author's name, and 'top'. Color illustrations are reproduced at the author's expense.

References: In the text identify references by Arabic numerals [in square brackets]. Material submitted for publication but not yet accepted should be noted as 'unpublished data' and not be included in the reference list. The list of references should include only those publications which are cited in the text. Do not alphabetize; number references in the order in which they are first mentioned in the text. The surnames of the authors followed by initials should be given. There should be no punctuation other than a comma to separate the authors. Cite all authors, 'et al' is not sufficient. Abbreviate journal names according to the Index Medicus system. (Also see International Committee of Medical Journal Editors: Uniform requirements for manuscripts submitted to biomedical journals. Br Med J 1988;296:401–405.)

Examples

(a) Papers published in periodicals: Kauffman HF, van der Heide S, Beaumont F, Blok H, de Vries K: Class-specific antibody determination against *Aspergillus fumigatus* by means of the enzyme-linked immunosorbent assay. III. Comparative study: IgG, IgA, IgM ELISA titers, precipitating antibodies and IgE binding after fractionation of the antigen. Int Arch Allergy Appl Immunol 1986;80:300–306.

(b) Monographs: Matthews DE, Farewell VT: Using and Understanding Medical Statistics. Basel, Karger, 1985.

(c) Edited books: Hardy WD Jr, Essex M: FeLV-induced feline acquired immune deficiency syndrome: A model for human AIDS; in Klein E (ed): Acquired Immunodeficiency Syndrome. Prog Allergy. Basel, Karger, 1986, vol 37, pp 353–376.

Full address: The exact postal address complete with postal code of the senior author must be given. If correspondence is handled by someone else, indicate this accordingly.

Further details: Authors may consult our leaflet 'Rules for the Preparation of Manuscripts', available on request from the Publisher, S. Karger AG, P.O. Box, CH–4009 Basel (Switzerland).

Page charges: There is no page charge for papers of 6 or fewer printed pages (including tables, illustrations and references). Each additional complete or partial page is charged to the author at SFr. 225.– / US $ 150.00. The allotted size of a paper is equal to approx. 12 manuscript pages (including tables, illustrations and references).

Galley proofs: Unless indicated otherwise, galley proofs are sent to the first-named author and should be returned with the least possible delay. Alterations made in galley proofs, other than the correction of printer's errors, are charged to the author. No page proofs are supplied.

Reprints: Order forms and a price list are sent with the galley proofs. Orders submitted after the issue is printed are subject to considerably higher prices. Allow five weeks from date of publication for delivery of reprints .

KARGER

Methods and Achievements in Experimental Pathology
(ISSN 0076-681-X), **Vol. 14**
Series Editor: G. Jasmin, Montréal, Qué.

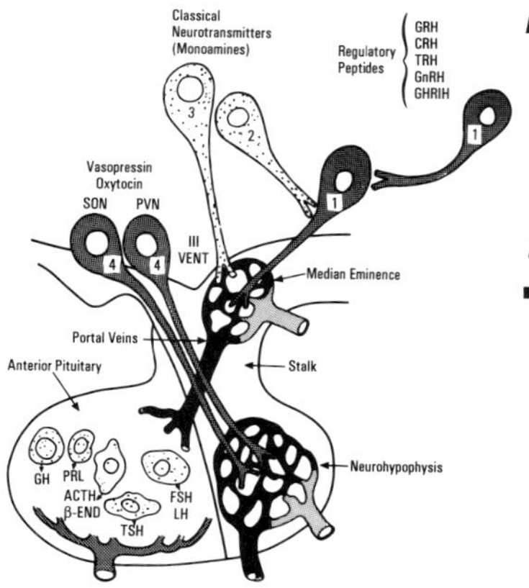

Editors: G. Jasmin, M. Cantin

Stress Revisited

I. Neuroendocrinology of Stress

New techniques in molecular biology have enabled the isolation of numerous peptides now recognized as playing key roles in the stress response. This unique two-volume work, consisting of invited contributions by prominent researchers in the field, represents an extensive survey of stress research at the present time. Volume 1 focuses on the neuroendocrine mediation of stress. Following clear coverage of the anatomy of the hypothalamic-pituitary axis, the participation of corticotropin-releasing factor and opioid peptides in the stress response is outlined. The next two articles discuss the effects of stress on cytokine production and the role of interleukins in the stress response. Further contributions consider stress and catecholamines, corticosteroid receptors and homeostasis, and finally, the neuroendocrine and pharmacological mechanisms of stress.

Updating basic knowledge of stress mediators with implications in biology and medicine, this thoroughly referenced text will greatly interest neuroscientists, endocrinologists, pathologists, and therapists in psychiatry or the behavioral sciences.

Contents

Pelletier, G. (Ste-Foy, P.Q.): Anatomy of the Hypothalamic-Pituitary Axis · *De Souza, E.B.; Grigoriadis, D.E.; Webster, E.L.* (Baltimore, Md.): Role of Brain, Pituitary and Spleen Corticotropin-Releasing Factor Receptors in the Stress Response · *Abraham, E.* (Los Angeles, Calif.): Effects of Stress on Cytokine Production · *Rivier, C.* (La Jolla, Calif.): Role of Interleukins in the Stress Response · *Kuchel, O.* (Montréal, P.Q.): Stress and Catecholamines · *de Kloet, E.R.; Joëls, M.; Oitzl, M.; Sutanto, W.* (Leiden/Utrecht): Implication of Brain Corticosteroid Receptor Diversity for the Adaptation Syndrome Concept · *Van de Kar, L.D.; Richardson-Morton, K.D.; Rittenhouse, P.A.* (Maywood, Ill.): Stress: Neuroendocrine and Pharmacological Mechanisms

Companion Volume
Methods and Achievements in Experimental Pathology, Vol. 15
Stress Revisited
2. Systemic Effects of Stress
Editors: Jasmin, G.; Proschek, L. (Montréal, Qué.)
approx. XVI + 224 p., 34 fig., 10 tab., hard cover, 1991
SFr. 248.– / DM 297.– / £ 107.90 / US$ 198.50
US$ price for USA, £ price for UK only (subject to change)
ISBN 3-8055-5403-X

Complete Set: Vol. 14 + 15
Stress Revisited
SFr. 399.– / DM 478.– / £ 173.50 / US$ 319.25
ISBN 3-8055-5404-4

Fields of Interest

Pathology; Neurology; Natural Sciences for Physicians; Behavioral Research, Biology for Physicians, Endocrinology, Molecular Biology, Neuroendocrinology, Psychiatry

Methods and Achievements in Experimental Pathology, Vol. 14
Stress Revisited
1. Neuroendocrinology of Stress
Editors: Jasmin, G.; Cantin, M. (Montréal, Qué.)
XII + 176 p., 34 fig., 5 tab., hard cover, 1991
SFr. 195.– / DM 234.– / £ 84.80 / US$ 156.00
US$ price for USA, £ price for UK only (subject to change)
ISBN 3-8055-5374-9

KI 91555

KARGER

Methods and Achievements in Experimental Pathology
(ISSN 0076-681-X), **Vol. 15**
Series Editor: G. Jasmin, Montréal, Qué.

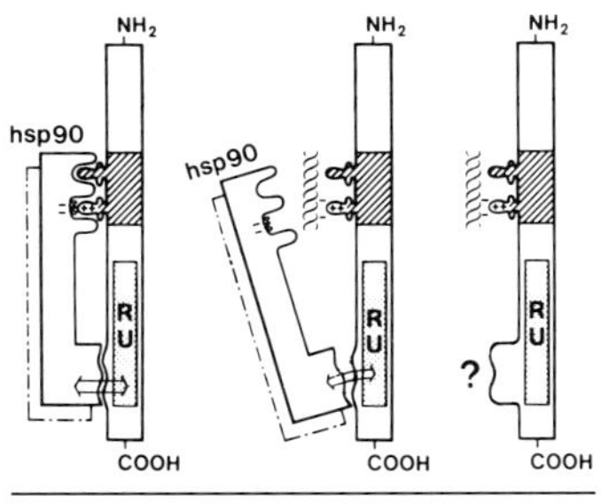

Three mechanisms

Editors: G. Jasmin, L. Proschek

Stress Revisited

2. Systemic Effects of Stress

The concept of stress has evolved from one based on stimulus-induced organic responses to one emphasizing the experience of stress and the handling of stressful information. This unique two-volume work, consisting of invited contributions by prominent researchers in the field, represents an extensive survey of stress research at the present time. Volume 2 focuses primarily on the systemic effects of stress. Following a stimulating discussion of the major mechanisms of stress, further articles describe in detail the systemic effects of stress on blood pressure, on the heart, as well as on learning and memory. In addition, the effects of stress at the molecular and cellular level, particularly the induction of stress proteins, are elucidated. The final contribution explores the role of stressful life events in affective disorders.
Contributing to a better understanding of the physiological and psychological consequences of stress, this text will greatly interest neuroscientists, endocrinologists, pathologists, and therapists in psychiatry or the behavioral sciences concerned with this very complex biological phenomenon.

Contents

Laborit, H. (Paris): The Major Mechanisms of Stress · *Hamet, P.; Malo, D.; Tremblay, J.* (Montréal, P.Q.): Genetic Basis of Increased Sensitivity to Environmental Stress in Hypertension · *Pasternac, A.; Talajic, M.* (Montréal, P.Q.): The Effects of Stress, Emotion, and Behavior on the Heart · *Hansen, M.; Rupp, H.* (Tübingen): Cellular and Molecular Changes in the Heart during Stress or Exercise · *Rappaport, L.; Contard, F.; Dubus, I.; Swynghedauw, B.; Samuel, J.L.* (Paris): Stress-Induced Proto-Oncogenes in the Myocardium · *Baulieu, E.-E.* (Bicêtre): The Connection between Steroid Receptors and Stress Protein (hsp90) · *Black, A.R.; Subjeck, J.R.* (Buffalo, N.Y.): The Biology and Physiology of the Heat Shock and Glucose-Regulated Stress Protein Systems · *De Wied, D.; Croiset, G.* (Utrecht): Stress Modulation of Learning and Memory Processes · *Serban, G.* (New York, N.Y.): Stress in Affective Disorders

Companion Volume
Methods and Achievements in Experimental Pathology, Vol. 14
Stress Revisited
1. Neuroendocrinology of Stress
Editors: Jasmin, G.;
Cantin, M. (Montréal, Qué.)
XII + 176 p., 34 fig., 5 tab.,
hard cover, 1991
SFr. 195.– / DM 234.– / £ 84.80 /
US$ 156.00
US$ price for USA, £ price for UK only (subject to change)
ISBN 3-8055-5374-9

Complete Set: Vol. 14 + 15
Stress Revisited
SFr. 399.– / DM 478.– / £ 173.50 /
US$ 319.25
ISBN 3-8055-5404-4

Fields of Interest
Pathology; Neurology; Natural Sciences for Physicians; Behavioral Research, Biology for Physicians, Endocrinology, Molecular Biology, Neuroendocrinology, Psychiatry

Methods and Achievements in Experimental Pathology, Vol. 15
Stress Revisited
2. Systemic Effects of Stress
Editors: Jasmin, G.; Proschek, L. (Montréal, Qué.)
approx. XVI + 224 p., 34 fig., 10 tab., hard cover, 1991
SFr. 248.– / DM 297.– / £ 107.90 / US$ 198.50
US$ price for USA, £ price for UK only (subject to change)
ISBN 3-8055-5403-X

KARGER

The Psychopathology of Perception

Proceedings of the Third Leeds Psychopathology Symposium September 29–30, 1988

Guest Editors
A.M. Mortimer, Leeds
K.J.B. Rix, Leeds

5 figures, 7 tables, 1991

KARGER

The Leeds Psychopathology Symposia

The Department of Psychiatry of the University of Leeds has held a Psychopathology Symposium every 2 years since 1984.

The recent psychopathology tradition in Leeds goes back to the period during which the late Professor Max Hamilton edited the influential 'Fish's Clinical Psychopathology: Signs and Symptoms in Psychiatry' and pioneered measurement in psychiatry.

Following in that tradition, Leeds continues to be particularly associated with psychopathology through 'Symptoms in the Mind', which is written by Hamilton's successor, Professor Andrew Sims and through further research into measurement in psychiatry under the direction of Dr. R.P. Snaith.

The symposia held to date have been:

The Psychopathology of Depression 1984
The Psychopathology of Body Image 1986
The Psychopathology of Perception 1988
The Psychopathology of Delusions and Awareness of Reality 1990

The proceedings of the 1986 symposium were published as a supplement to the *British Journal of Psychiatry* and the proceedings of the 1990 symposium are being processed for publication. The next symposium will be on the Psychopathology of Speech.

Keith J.B. Rix, University of Leeds

S. Karger · Medical and Scientific Publishers
Basel · München · Paris · London · New York · New Delhi · Bangkok · Singapore · Tokyo · Sydney

Drug Dosage
The authors and the publisher have exerted every effort to ensure that drug selection and dosage set forth in this text are in accord with current recommendations and practice at the time of publication. However, in view of ongoing research, changes in government regulations, and the constant flow of information relating to drug therapy and drug reactions, the reader is urged to check the package insert for each drug for any change in indications and dosage and for added warnings and precautions. This is particularly important when the recommended agent is a new and/or infrequently employed drug.

Printed in Switzerland on acid-free paper by
Thür AG Offsetdruck, Pratteln
ISBN 3-8055-5536-9

Psychopathology 1991;24:347–355

0254–4962/91/0246–0347$2.75/0

The Duphar Lecture: On the Etiology of Alien, Nonself Attributes of Schizophrenic 'Voices'

Ralph E. Hoffman

Yale University School of Medicine, New Haven, Conn., USA

Abstract. The etiology of schizophrenic hallucinations or 'voices' remains unknown. The following is a discussion of a hypothesis linking these hallucinatory phenomena to a disruption in discourse planning. The relationship between normal imagery and hallucination is discussed. The concept of 'alien intentionality' is introduced, and a theoretical argument is presented which links this phenomenon with the exteriorization of internal images. Statistical data linking discourse planning disruptions and schizophrenic data are reviewed, and a description of the treatment of a hallucinating schizophrenic via a novel type of speech therapy is described.

The purpose of this report is to extend and elaborate upon an earlier discussion [Hoffman, 1986a, b] pertaining to the nature and etiology of schizophrenic hallucinations. The views presented below combine the perspectives of psychopathology research, cognitive science, and neuroscience.

Schizophrenic hallucinations tend to be reported as auditory, and, by and large, are described by the patients themselves as 'voices'. Many schizophrenic patients also report hallucinations in other modalities. However, a study of schizophrenic patients in New York City indicated that those patients with visual hallucinations inevitably experience auditory hallucinations; the reverse was not the case – many patients with auditory hallucinations did not suffer from visual hallucinations [Alpert, 1986]. Along these same lines, a cross-cultural report has indicated that although schizophrenics in non-Western cultures may be prone to experiencing visual hallucinations, these patients experience auditory hallucinations as well [Al-Issa, 1977]. Thus hallucinations of the auditory type seem more or less to be a common demoninator among hallucinating schizophrenics.

The phenomenology of normal mental imagery is of central importance in understanding the nature of hallucination. Our experience of our own 'thoughts' or 'consciousness' is often composed of mental images [Hoffman and Kravitz, 1987]. With little to no effort, one can produce internal visual images, for instance, of a tree or one's grandmother. These internal images of objects or scenes seem to have 'sensory' properties such as color and shape [Kossyln, 1980]. Similarly, one also can willfully induce auditory images having 'sensory' properties such as tone, timbre and loudness which have a particular temporal sequence. In this fashion, one can create an internal auditory image of automobile horns honking, or the final choral movement of Beethoven's Ninth Symphony. The voices of schizophrenic patients also have auditory imagery characteristics. The voices 'sound' either male or female, speak softly, loudly, with a certain pitch, etc. It seems beyond question that most auditory hallucinations are images having the sensory qualities of spoken speech.

A particularly frequent type of auditory image for most adults is the auditory image of one's own voice. We say words inwardly to ourselves all of the time. The importance of this 'inner speech' was first highlighted by Vygotsky [1932, 1978]. Vygotsky noted in his developmental studies of normal children that inner speech derives from outer speech. First the child learns to speak to others. Then he begins talking out loud to himself. This egocentric speech seems to play an important role in helping to guide the actions of the child during play and problem solving. Ultimately this egocentric speech is no longer spoken out loud but is nonetheless created as an internal imagistic 'voice' which the child and later the adult uses to guide, coax, cajole himself etc.

Just as we are able to produce an auditory verbal image of our own voice we can spontaneously create auditory images of other speakers. These auditory images have sensory qualities in the same sense that auditory images of music or automobile horns do.

This immediately raises the central question – what makes the 'voices' of schizophrenics different from the normal 'voice' of conscious mentation?

The most obvious answer to this question is that a schizophrenic 'voice' is an auditory image of an utterance whose acoustic properties are distinct from the subject's own voice. However, we can intentionally create internal auditory images of other speakers just as easily as we can create the internal visual image of a tree. Moreover, a study by Sedman [1966] has clearly indicated that at least some schizophrenic 'voices' consist of the subject's own voice.

A traditional perceptual defect model for schizophrenic voices assumed that sensory attributes such as exceptional loudness, vividness, or clarity cause certain verbal images to be identified as deviant. That loudness or vividness cannot be the critical variable is readily established simply by talking to hallucinating schizophrenics. Many will admit that their voices are at times barely audible – yet the experience is still hallucinatory in nature [Bleuler, 1950]. Another approach would be to propose that schizophrenic 'voices' are characterized by being exteriorized; however Sedman [1966] has argued that 'voices' can be experienced as alien and hallucinated even when experienced inside the head, a conclusion that was supported by a more recent systematic study by Junginger and Frame [1985]. The latter surveyed 52 hallucinating subjects, most of whom were schizophrenic, and were not able to identify any sensory feature including exteriorization, as a criterion that distinguishes hallucination from ordinary imagery.

This was confirmed by myself when I requested a small number of schizophrenics to reimagine a previous verbal hallucination in the present [Hoffman, 1986a]. They were then asked to contrast the two experiences in terms of loudness, vividness, etc. Invariably the subjects reported that the reimaginings were different from true 'voices', but were not generally able to identify any particular sensory qualities that distinguished the two. Generally the subjects reported that the reimagined voice sounded the same – but that there remained a difference – namely that in the second case the image 'came from me', while in the first case it did not.

Finally it is important to note that workers, in spite of extraordinary efforts dating back as far as 1952, have not been able to demonstrate that imagery production capabilities are consistently altered in schizophrenics [for review see Hoffman, 1986]. Thus I was led to question what besides these sensory qualities and perceptual processes could contribute to the hallucinatory attributes of schizophrenic 'voices'.

Internal images, while sharing sensory features of percepts derived from the 'outside world', are distinct from percepts in a critical way – they can be willfully induced: I can decide to image a tree and the tree will simply appear. Similarly I can intend to hear my father's voice and the voice is created as an auditory image. In short, images, while being percept-like, are also action-like.

Just as action and imaging can be intended or willed, so can certain actions (such as nervous tics) and speech (such as slips of the tongue) be experienced as unintended. Images can also be experienced as unintended; an obvious example is ordinary dreaming. The dream is generally experienced as completely out of control of the dreamer – it is perforce a hallucination.

This raises the question of whether a core component of the 'alien' experience of hallucination for the schizophrenic is that the image is experienced as involuntary – as occurring beyond the control of the subject. My small experiment requesting schizophrenics to intentionally reimagine a hallucination never caused a hallucination to be produced – thus suggesting that intentionally induced images are never experienced as hallucinations. Does this mean that unintendedness is *sufficient* to cause an image to be experienced as alien or nonself, i.e., a hallucination?

I believe not. Consider the following: Suppose you were on the highway driving in your car and you had a flat tire. You get out of the car and begin to change the tire. Now suppose while you are changing the tire, you developed an involuntary nervous twitch in your shoulder. This may be alarming, but certainly would not constitute an experience that would make one feel possessed by an alien force. Thus the involuntariness of an action does not necessarily cause one to experience the action as alien or nonself.

But now instead suppose that as you reached for the tire, your right hand involuntarily shot up in the air and started waving at the cars going by, thereby preventing you from changing the tire. My prediction is that this experience would be quite a bit more alarming – as if an alien, nonself force had taken possession of your arm. This prediction is supported by a very interesting stroke syndrome studied by Goldberg [1985]. These patients suffer from lesions of the supplementary motor area of the frontal lobes; this cortical area has been identified as being central to the initiation of purposeful motoric actions. These patients develop 'alien hands' which seem to have acquired purposes of their own that are out of control of the subject. For instance, the hand may attempt to unbutton clothing when the subject has no intention of doing so. This rare form of stroke can produce a kind of psychosis. Some of these patients, none of whom have prior histories of psychiatric disturbance [Goldberg, personal commun.], came to believe that their arms had been possessed by alien, nonself forces.

Goals are essential in generating intelligent behavior. Workers in artificial intelligence have shown that even modest attempts to simulate intelligent sequential behavior using computer programs requires the representation of a goal and a set of subgoals and plans that are designed to carry out the goal [Schank and Abelson, 1977; Sacerdoti, 1977]. In real life, goal-driven planning processes often occur outside of conscious awareness. Consider for example the process whereby I go to work in the morning. I have in mind, though am not thinking about it overly much, the goal of going to work. As a result of that overarching goal, a hierarchy of subgoals are generated – e.g. transporting myself to my car, driving car to work, leaving car and entering hospital, etc. Each one of these subgoals has its own set lower level goals. For instance, in terms of leaving car and entering the hospital, I must park car, turn off ignition, extract myself from the seat, etc. The hierarchy of goals, subgoals, and motoric plans that realize all of these hundreds of subgoals are somehow represented in a psychologically real sense.

Goals and subgoals subtending routine motoric actions are ordinarily realized and coordinated in effortless fashion. A nervous tic feels involuntary because it does not reflect a motoric plan consonant with the current goal of the organism. But it is not experienced as 'nonself' because it does not express a goal. In contrast, our hypothetical example of involuntary handwaving while attempting to change a tire and the 'alien hands' described by Goldberg [1985] express a motoric plan that is experienced as intentional in the sense that it refers to a particular goal. However, it is an 'alien intentionality' because goals which are autonomous with respect to the conscious mentation of the subject are expressed and elaborated upon [Brand, 1986]. In a parallel fashion I propose that 'voices' correspond to internal auditory images of speech whose content expresses autonomous goals, and hence, their own 'alien intentionality'.

Research in psycholinguistics has suggested that, just as in the case of motoric actions, a speaker normally generates a hierarchically organized plan that accomplishes the communicative goals and subgoals of the speaker [Deese, 1978; van Dijk, 1980]. This plan is then transformed into an actual string of spoken sentences. Without this preliminary discourse plan, the speaker could not utilize multiple sentences of clauses in a coordinated fashion to express a coherent message.

Schizophrenics often produce incoherent language [Chaika, 1981, 1982; Reilly et al., 1975; Andreasen, 1979a, b]. This suggests that those cognitive processes producing discourse plans which establish and elaborate upon communication goals may be disturbed for many schizophrenic patients; textual analysis of schizophrenic utterances has strongly suggested that this indeed is the case [Hoffman et al., 1982, Hoffman, 1986a]. Two examples of poorly planned schizophrenic texts are [Hoffman, 1986a, for more extensive analysis]:

(I) Interviewer: Did you ever try to hurt yourself? (patient being asked about her suicidality after being admitted to a psychiatric hospital)

Patient: I cut myself once when I was in the kitchen trying to please David. I was scared for (sic) life because David didn't want me and if David didn't want me then no man would.

(II) Interviewer: Tell me about (your experiences in) school?

Patient: School? Well there are schools of play and schools of fish, mostly you see fish school, people edumacating (sic) themselves, you see, sea is one thing and education is another. Fish is school in their community, that's why the community of man stands in the way of the community of the sea, and once they see the light of sunny sunshine then they well let it be...

Compare (I) and (II) with the following:

(III) Interviewer: Can you describe where you live?

Patient: Yes, I live in Connecticut. We live in a fifty year old Tudor house. It's a house that's very much a home ... ah ... I live there with my husband and son. It's a home where people are drawn to feel comfortable, walk in, let's see ... a home that is furnished comfortably – not expensive – a home that shows very much my personality.

Segment (I) suggests a condensation of two disjoint communication goals. One is the attempt to describe an incident where the speaker accidently cuts herself. In this context, 'I was scared for life' seems to refer to her reaction to seeing that she had accidentally cut herself. A second communication goal is to directly respond to the issue of her own potential suicidality when she generates statements such as 'no man would (want me)' and 'David doesn't want me'. Segment (II) corresponds to more haphazard conflation of multiple communication goals that may include the goal of describing the negative effects of man on nature ('the community of man versus the community of sea'), the fact that the word 'school' possesses different meanings, that both men and animals have 'schools', etc. In contrast, segment (III) has an obvious conversional goal that organizes the entire utterance, namely to describe aspects of the speaker's personality in terms of her home and her family.

As described above, Vygotsky [1932, 1978] has postulated that the cognitive processes leading to the verbal images of inner speech are largely the same as that which produces outward speech. If schizophrenics produce overt speech plans serving multiple inconsistent conversational goals, then their internal verbal imagery may at times reflect disparate communication goals and plans. If these verbal images clash with the dominant conscious goals of the subject, they would be experienced as involuntary and if they express whole sentences that have their own 'alien intentionality' the experience could be very noxious and disturbing for the subject.

This formulation predicts that the more a schizophrenic is subject to discourse planning breakdowns, the more likely it is that he is to experience verbal hallucinations. This hypothesis was supported by an analysis of discourse planning applied to psychotic speech [Hoffman 1986]. Schizophrenics with and without verbal hallucinations were compared in terms of the severity of their discourse planning disturbance. Mean scores of severity of planning disturbance was approximately three times as great in the former group compared with the latter, a result that was statistically significant to the $p < 0.005$ level.

The first question that can be asked about such correlational data is whether the finding was due to the fact that the hallucinating patients were simply sicker overall – therefore having more positive symptoms and language difficulties [Faber, 1986, Schwartz, 1986]. This was checked by examining discourse deviance scores in schizophrenics who had delusions and those who did not. If the effect noted was due simply to overall severity of illness, then a similar correspondence should turn up for this symptom. Statistically speaking, the correlations between severity of delusions and discourse planning scores was very close to zero – suggesting some specificity in terms of the relationship between discourse planning deviance and verbal hallucinations.

A second question that can be raised is: Why is it that the overt speech of schizophrenics is not experienced more often as alien and of nonself origin? The answer is quite simple – when a person is speaking out loud he has prima facie evidence that he is doing the speaking – regardless of content – this due to the proprioceptive sensations of muscle activity of tongue, lips and larynx during speech production. In contrast, inner speech lacks self-confirming conscious proprioceptive sensation. Even though some trace EMG activity is detectable during inner speech [Sokolov, 1972], this muscle activity is not robust enough to induce a conscious motoric experience.

A third question relates to the fact that many occurrences of schizophrenic 'voices' are perceived as deriving from an exterior, nonself space cast in a nonfirst-person voice. How might certain involuntarily produced verbal images acquire such attributes? A clue is another mental exercise: Visually imagine a striped, four legged animal. Few of us would imagine a striped cow, but would tend to imagine tigers or zebras. We produce imagery experiences in the present on the basis of expectations derived from our past experience. Striped animals that we know are tigers and zebras, not cows. Similarly, when we experience involuntarily produced auditory/verbal images which express 'autonomous' communicative intentions departing from our current goals, the ordinary expectation, based on a lifetime of experience, is that these are voices of other speakers outside of the head. As in the case of the striped animal example, the cognitive apparatus of the schizophrenic will create the consequent image that conforms to its attributes, in this case that the verbal message expresses alien, unintended goals. The otherwise intact cognitive apparatus of the schizophrenic will be prone to cast these imagery experiences in a nonself voice projected into an exteriorized, nonself space.

One might respond to this argument by noting that the exteriorization of auditory perceptual experiences seems to be 'hard-wired'. In higher mammals auditory information is mapped out as a spatial receptive field in the contralateral temporal lobe [Masterson and Imig, 1984; Jenkins and Merzenich, 1981]. It seems counterintuitive that such hard-wired cortical representations could be stimulated by something as ephemeral as an expectation. However, just because something is neurally coded at a primary sensory level does not mean that it is not penetrable by cognitive expectations. For instance, a study by von der Heydt et al. [1984] demonstrated that certain visual illusions can induce firing of area 18 visual cortical neurons in monkeys even when their receptive fields are not being stimulated. Although this physiological study pertained to visual and not verbal imagery expectations, it does strongly support the hypothesis that in general cognitive expectations can and do alter firing patterns in primary sensory receptive areas, and that the neurally coded 'exteriorization' of verbal images by cognitive expectation – and the induction of a 'true' hallucination – is entirely possible.

An additional and appropriate criticism of my model is that some schizophrenics with verbal hallucinations seem not to demonstrate discourse deviance. My belief, however, is that schizophrenics can compensate for their discourse planning difficulties. One method is to stick to rather simple speech productions. Our earlier work analyzing the discourse structure of psychotic speech suggested a threshold effect. If the complexity of communicative intentions remains under threshold, coherence can be maintained even if the individual suffers from discourse planning defects – when discourse complexity exceeds threshold, incoherence results. A second compensatory devise for schizophrenics is rehearsal. Many schizophrenics have rehearsed scripts which they repeat exceedingly well; frequently these scripts are their paranoid ideas. But when requested to talk about something unrehearsed, they quickly get into trouble.

In order to test out these ideas, I decided to work intensively with one of these exceptional cases: a schizophrenic woman who was plagued with voices which were refractory to all forms of treatment for numerous years, yet, for the most part, her speech was coherent. I wanted to determine three things: (1) Were this woman's discourse planning abilities indeed intact? If so, a theory of schizophrenic 'voices' based on discourse planning disturbances would be essentially disproved. (2) If she did demonstrate impaired discourse planning, were these impairments at least partially remediable using targeted speech therapy techniques? (3) If remediation of discourse planning defects was achieved, would her voices be reduced? If so, this would provide further support for the hypothesis. In terms of (1), my suspicions were confirmed. The patient could certainly speak coherently, but this was only about a standard set of topics where she lamented about her illness, the wrongs done to her by her family, etc. As soon as I requested her to depart from these topics she would be able to speak fluently for a short while but then, invariably, a complete blockage of speech would develop. It turned out that this difficulty recurred frequently. Subjectively speaking, she described the blockage as a process whereby she is caught in an ever narrowing tunnel, crushed by the multiplicity of her own ideas. Inevitably, these instances were followed by voices. Generally these voices were critical of her and were both inside and outside of her head. When outside, she tended to hear them on her right side.

My attempts to provide treatment began by my explaining to her my way of understanding the cause of her voices – that they derived from the fact that her attempts to speak triggered off an excessive number of different things to say which are out of her control and then get expressed as voices. I told her that the key task was to help her sort out the different things that she had in mind to say so that they all could be expressed coherently, and that we really needed to focus on her blockages since those were the times that she seemed most overwhelmed by competing things to say. Consequently we developed a strategy where she would 'talk through' her blockages using a tape recorder. The results generally demonstrated discourse incoherence and multiple competing ideas. These different fragments were then written down on slips of paper and she practiced reconstructing them into coherent paragraphs. We also played a card game – I had gone through a Thesaurus and pulled out, at random, a large number of words and phrases. Then I had her practice, first using 2 cards and later building up to 6 cards, constructing in speech a paragraph that was well organized and incorporated what was stated in the cards. All of her responses were tape-recorded, so she had a chance to listen to herself speak and correct her incoherent speech productions. After 6 weeks of this work her voices stopped, the first time in many years. Since then she had a partial recurrence after treatment terminated; however, the recurrence has not been as intense as a preteatment baseline.

No firm conclusions can be drawn from this work – this was a single case, and the treatment did not have a permanent curative effect. It seems as if the patient needed to continue to practice these language exercises in order to retain her gains. Also it cannot be ruled out that the reduction in voices was secondary to a placebo effect. However, it is striking that this 'linguistically coherent' hallucinating schizophrenic speaker could be induced to demonstrate considerable discourse incoherence under the proper conditions, and that the frequency of voices seem to be reduced by efforts to correct her speech blockage – which she herself described as being the result of a conflation of multiple speech intentions.

What etiology can be proposed for the type of the language production disturbance described above? Many schizophrenic patients have demonstrated pathological reductions in cerebral metabolism in frontal areas [Buchsbaum and Haier, 1987]. This could be directly relevant to discourse planning disturbances since it is likely that the prefrontal cortex is the initiator and goal-setter of propositional speech [Goldberg, 1985]. Thus one could postulate that higher order message planning during language production in schizophrenia may be disrupted by a disturbance of functioning in the prefrontal cortex.

In summary, the model of verbal hallucinations that I propose is consonant with Brown's [1987] belief that neurological symptoms in general are not produced by the lesion itself, but by the cognitive output of the remaining intact tissue in response to the lesion. Along these lines I hypothesize that the imagery production apparatus is quite intact in schizophrenia. Instead the 'lesion' involves language production processes producing messages with autonomous goals. This is responded to by an intact imagery production apparatus through assignment of nonself attributes to the verbal image. These nonself attributes are derived from the ordinary verbal imagery expectations of speech produced by others, i.e., the verbal messages which ordinarily expresses autonomous goals.

Even if this hypothesis turns out to be incorrect, this discussion hopefully illustrates the usefulness of intervention studies. I do not believe that any etiological theory of hallucinations in schizophrenia can be established by any particular cognitive or physiological test alone. This is because these research strategies can only yield correlational data which never establish the direction of causality. The challenge is to develop targeted interventions that specifically modify the purported cognitive or physiological defect – and then to determine if there is a parallel shift in psychopathology.

References

Al-Issa, I.: Social and cultural aspects of hallucinations. Psychol. Bull. *84:* 570–587 (1977).

Alpert, M.: Language process and hallucination phenomenology. Behav. Brain Sci. *9:* 518–519 (1986).

Andreasen, N.C.: Thought, language and communication disorders: 1. Clinical assessment, definition of terms, and evaluation of their reliability. Archs gen. Psychiat. *36:* 1315–1321 (1979a).

Andreasen, N.C.: Thought, language and communication disorders: 2. Diagnostic significance. Archs gen. Psychiat. *36:* 1325–1330 (1979b).

Bleuler, E.: Dementia praecox or the group of schizophrenias. (International University Press, New York 1950).

Brand, M.: Intended versus intentional action. Behav. Brain Sci. *9:* 520–521 (1986).

Brown, J.W.: The life of the mind (IRBN Press, New York 1987).

Buchsbaum, M.S.; Haier, R.J.: Functional and anatomical brain imaging: impact on schizophrenia research. Schiz. Bull. *13:* 115–132 (1987).

Chaika, E.: How shall a discourse be understood? Disc. Proc. *4:* 71–88 (1981).

Chaika, E.: A unified explanation for the diverse structural deviations reported for adult schizophrenics with disrupted speech. J. Commun. Disord. *15:* 167–189 (1982).

Deese, J.: Thought into speech. Am. Scient. *66:* 314–321 (1978).

Faber, R.: The diversity of the schizophrenias. Behav. Brain Sci. *9:* 522 (1986).

Goldberg, G.: Supplementary motor area structure and function: Review and hypotheses. Behav. Brain Sci. *8:* 567–616 (1985).

Hoffman, R.E.: Apprehending schizophrenic discourse: the listener's task re-examined. Brain Lang. *15:* 207–233 (1982).

Hoffman, R.E.: What can schizophrenic 'voices' tell us? Behav. Brain Sci. *9:* 535–548 (1986a).

Hoffman, R.E.: Verbal hallucinations and language production processes in schizophrenia. Behav. Brain Sci. *9:* 503–548 (1986b).

Hoffman, R.E.; Kravitz, R.E.: Feedforward action regulation and the experience of will. Behav. Brain Sci. *10:* 782–783 (1987).

Jenkins, W.M.; Merzenich, M.M.: Lesions of restricted frequency representational sectors within primary auditory cortex produce frequency dependent sound localization defects. Soc. Neurosci. Abstr. *7:* 392 (1981).

Junginger, J.J.; Frame, C.L.: Self-report of the frequency and phenomenology of verbal hallucinations. J. Nerv. Ment. Dis. *173:* 149–150 (1985).

Kossyln, S.M.: Image and mind (Harvard University Press, Cambridge 1980).

Masterson, R.B.; Imig, T.J.: Neural mechanisms for sound localization. A. Rev. Physiol. *46:* 275–287 (1984).

Reilly, F.; Harrow, M.; Tucker, G.; Quinlan, D.; Siegel, A.: Looseness of associations in acute schizophrenia. Br. J. Psychiat. *127:* 24–46 (1975).

Sacerdoti, E.D.: A structure for plans and behavior (Elsevier, New York 1977).

Schank, R.; Abelson, R.: Scripts, plans, goals, and understanding (Erlbaum, Hillsdale 1977).

Schwartz, S.: Hallucination, rationalization, and response set. Behav. Brain Sci. *9:* 532–533 (1986).

Sedman, G.: 'Inner voices': phenomenological and clinical aspects. Br. J. Psychiat. *112:* 485–490 (1966).

Sokolov, A.N.: Inner speech and thought (Plenum Press, New York 1972).

Van Dijk, T.: Macrostructures: an interdisciplinary study of global structures in discourse, interaction, and cognition (Erlbaum, Hillsdale 1980).

Von der Heydt, R.; Peterhans, E.; Baumgartner, G.: Illusory contours and cortical neuron responses. Science *224:* 1260–1262 (1984).

Vygotsky, L.S.: Thought in schizophrenia. Archs Neurol. Psychiat. *31:* 1063–1077 (1932).

Vygotsky, L.S.: Mind in society: The development of higher psychological processes (Harvard University Press, Cambridge 1978).

Ralph E. Hoffman, MD
Yale University School of Medicine
Box 12A Yale Station
New Haven, CT 06520 (USA)

Psychopathology 1991;24:356–360

0254–4962/91/0246–0356$2.75/0

Musical Hallucinations: A Statistical Analysis of 46 Cases

G.E. Berrios

Department of Psychiatry, University of Cambridge, Addenbrooke's Hospital, Cambridge, UK

Abstract. Musical hallucinations remain rare, are more common in women, and their onset is often related to ear pathology, particularly deafness. When brain disease is involved, pathology of the right or non-dominant hemisphere seems overrepresented. Psychosis and personality traits play a minimal role in their development. A discriminant function was constructed that correctly predicted the presence of brain disease (89%) and included the following clinical variables: being male, having acute onset musical hallucinations, and absence of deafness, psychiatric disease, and other forms of hallucination.

The term 'musical hallucinations' describes the clinical phenomenon of hearing tunes and melodies which are not relevantly related to external stimuli [1,2]. The experience may be continuous or intermittent, and is often accompanied by insight. They are reported less often than other forms of auditory hallucinations [3, 4] or tinnitus [5]. They may be experienced in a variety of conditions including disease of the ear [6], neurological [7], and psychiatric pathology [8], and toxic states [9–11]. Depending on the aetiology, onset may be acute or gradual. They may be the only complaint or part of a constellation of acousmata which can 'mature' and become complex sound forms or tunes [12].

In the case of deaf individuals [13], musical hallucinations may disintegrate after a time, and become replaced by short and iterative musical phrases, like the noise made by a scratched record. In the case of strokes or depressive illness, and as the underlying pathology resolves, musical hallucinations tend to disappear.

Subjects and Methods

Up to 1989, there were about 135 cases of musical hallucinations in the literature. Only 36 contained sufficient clinical data for statistical analysis [list of references available from author]. To these 10 new ones have been added. These 46 cases constitute sample *Index 1*. The variables analyzed are shown in table 1.

Subjects with musical hallucinations who were also deaf (30 out of 46) were made into a sub-sample *(Index 2)*. Five control samples were studied: *Control 3:* 44 subjects with visual hallucinations [15]; *Control 4:* 90 subjects with presbyacusis; *Control 5:* 38 subjects with tinnitus; *Control 6:* 207 subjects with inner ear disease [16]; and *Control 7:* 21 subjects with visual hallucinations and advanced impairment of vision [15]. The sample of 69 cases with epilepsy and 'experimental' hallucinations reported by Penfield and Perot [7] was analyzed as 21 happened to have experienced musical hallucinations, either spontaneously or after cortical stimulation.

Results

Table 1 summarizes clinical features for the 46 cases. Noteworthy features are the marked predominance of females and the age of the group. Two-thirds were deaf. In 40% musical hallucinations were the only symptom. The latter were mainly subjects with strokes, tumours or epileptic foci, without deafness or psychiatric history. Songs, whether accompanied by instruments or not, were the most common form, religious and patriotic hymns being quite popular. Hallucinations tended, in general, to be heard most of the time, either as alternating tunes or as repeating musical phrase. Gradual fragmentation of melodies was seen in a fair number of patients, and there was a trend for this to correlate with duration of the disease. Insight (present from the start or soon gained) occurred in 73% of subjects. 73% of subjects had *no* psychiatric history (either past or concomitant). In the case of concomitant disease depression accounted for most of the variance. In 40% there was evidence of brain disease (table 2). Tables 3–5 show that subjects with musical hallucinations of acute onset tended not to be deaf but belonged in the group of tumours, strokes and epilepsy. Patients affected by ear disease tended to experience other forms of hallucinations, mainly tinnitus and humming, which had gradual onset. Those with brain disease tended to have insight; those with psychiatric disease did not. Tables 3–5 also show the results of an *exploratory* factor analysis of the Index 1 sample which extracted four factors: ENT, brain disease, psychiatric and musical. A discriminant function was then obtained which could classify correctly 89% of the sample as having 'brain disease'. It profiled subjects who were male,

Table 1. Musical hallucinations (n = 46)

Sex, F/M		37/9
Age	mean ± SD	60±19
	median	62
	mode	75
Lateralization	bilateral	31
	right	8
	left	7
Type of onset	acute	17
	gradual	29
Modifiable	yes/no	6/30
Predominant	instrumental	18
	singing	25
	animal singing	2
Insight	yes/no	33/13
Ear disease	present	29
	absent	16
Deafness	present	31
	absent	15
Other hallucinations	acousmata	16
	voices	11
	visual	3
	absent	18
Psychiatric disease	yes/no	12/34

Table 2. Musical hallucinations: associated brain pathology

Temporal lobe tumour	6	R/L 5/1
EEG temporal foci	5[1]	
Stroke	3	R/L 3/0
Neurosyphilis	2	
Subarachnoid haem.	1	
Localized 'atrophy'	1	
Behçet's syndrome	1	
Brain injury (RTA)	1	
Induced by ECT	1	
None found or reported	28	

[1] There was underlying pathology in 3 cases: stroke in 2 and tumour in 1.

Table 3. Musical hallucinations: significant intra-group correlations (n = 46)

	Age	Onset (acute)	Other hallucinations	Brain disease	Psychiatric disease
Deafness	0.46	-0.49		-0.49	
Ear disease			0.41		
Onset (gradual)			0.48	-0.47	
Insight				0.44	-0.51

All values $p < 0.01$ (Bonferroni corrected).

Table 4. Principal component analysis (n = 46; variables = 12)

Factor extracted	Eigenvalue	Cumulative variance, %
ENT	3	25
Brain disease	1.7	41
Psychiatric	1.4	54
Musical	1.3	66

Table 5. Discriminant function analysis (Wilks method; n = 46)

Discriminant function	Male No deafness Acute onset No psychiatric disease No other hallucination

Group variable: brain disease (present/absent).
DF correctly classifies 89% of cases ($p < 0.001$).

and had no deafness, musical hallucinations with acute onset, unaccompanied by any other form of hallucination, and no psychiatric disease.

Comparison of the two Index with the 5 Control samples showed that musically hallucinated patients were significantly younger than patients with visual hallucination, presbyacusis and tinnitus. There were more females amongst the subjects with musical hallucinations than amongst those with presbyacusis or tinnitus. The sample reported by Penfield and Perot [7] was younger and 30% had experienced at least one musical hallucination (only 42% had been spontaneous). A significant predominance of women (Fisher's exact test: $p < 0.05$) was also found when only the subjects who had experienced spontaneous musical hallucinations were considered.

Discussion and Conclusions

Caution must be exercised in the interpretation of data of mixed provenance. However, the sample reported here is probably the largest thus far and the variables analyzed were robust and reliable. The most salient findings have been that musical hallucinations seem to be more frequent in elderly females affected by deafness, or by brain disease, and with no history of psychiatric illness. It is important to rule out sampling artifacts (the female pool available to develop musical hallucinations is larger because females survive longer), or the intervention of mediating variables. However, age does not seem to be an important factor (no difference with presbyacusis or tinnitus). Furthermore, female predominance was also found in the much younger sample reported by Penfield and Perot [7]. With regard to the intervention of a mediating variable there is no evidence that epilepsy [17, 18], deafness [19], tinnitus [4, 20] or brain tumours [21–24] are more prevalent in females; nor that auditory hallucinations are more frequent in females with schizophrenia at any age [25, 26].

However, a predominance of females in a group of elderly individuals with visual hallucinations has been reported [15]. Thus females may experience (or report) hallucinations related to organic states more often than males. This conclusion cannot be extended, however, to hallucinations in general (i.e. voices in schizophrenia). It is unwarranted to speculate at this stage as to the mechanisms. Possibly females report their experiences more often, or the finding may reflect differences in lateralization [27, 28].

Other findings here confirm existing views that deafness [14], ear disease [29], advanced age [30], and brain disease [7] are important factors in the aetiology of auditory hallucinations. With regard to laterality, in the case of subjects with tumours, strokes or epileptic foci, the indication is that the non-dominant hemisphere seems to play an important role. This is consistent with what is known about music processing in the brain [31–34]. It also suggests a distinction between musical hallucinations and the putative mechanisms linked to hallucinatory voices in schizophrenia which seem related to the dominant hemisphere [35, 36]. With regard to differential diagnosis, occasionally, subjects with true palinacusis [37, 38], like the second case of Hécaen and Ropert [12], might be misdiagnosed as suffering from genuine musical hallucinations.

Acknowledgments

The author is grateful to Drs CU Cockshott, T Denning, and A West for allowing him to report 3 of their cases.

References

1 Ey, H.: Traité des hallucinations (Masson, Paris 1973).

2 Berrios, G.E.: Musical hallucinations: conceptual and historical aspects. Br. J. Psychiat. *156:* 188–194 (1990).

3 Berrios, G.E.: Hallucinosis; in Frederiks, Neurobehavioural disorders, pp. 565–572 (Elsevier, Amsterdam 1985).

4 Johnson, F.H.: The anatomy of hallucinations (Nelson Hall, Chicago 1978).

5 Berrios, G.E.; Rose, G.S.: Psychiatric aspects of tinnitus. Compreh. Psychiat. (submitted for publication).

6 Petazzi, A.: Contributo allo studio delle allucinazioni acustiche specialmente in rapporto con l'alterazione dell'apparato uditivo periferico. Archo ital. Otol. Rinol. Lar. *10:* 385–429 (1900).

7 Penfield, W.; Perot, P.: The brain's record of auditory and visual experience – a final summary and discussion. Brain *86:* 595–696 (1963).

8 Aizenberg, D.; Schwartz, B.; Modai, I.: Musical hallucinations, acquired deafness and depression. J. nerv. ment. Dis. *174:* 309–311 (1986).

9 Allen, J.R.: Salicylate-induced musical perceptions (letter). New Engl. J. Med. *313:* 642–643 (1985).

10 Victor, M.; Hope, J.M.: The phenomenon of auditory hallucinations in chronic alcoholism. J. nerv. ment. Dis. *126:* 451–481 (1958).

11 Malitz, S.; Wilkens, B.; Esecover, H.A.: Comparison of drug-induced hallucinations with those seen in spontaneously occurring psychoses; in

West, Hallucinations, pp. 50–63 (Grune & Stratton, New York 1962).
12 Hécaen, H.; Ropert, R.: Les hallucinations auditives des otopathes. J. Psychol. norm. path. *60:* 293–324 (1963).
13 Ross, E.D.; Jossman, P.B.; Bell, B.; Sabin, T.; Geschwind, N.: Musical hallucinations in deafness J. Am. Med. Ass. *231:* 620–621 (1975).
14 Régis, E.: Les hallucinations unilatérales et la pathologie des hallucinations. 7° Congrès des Aliénistes et Neurologistes de Langue Française, pp. 23–33 (Housseau, Nancy 1896).
15 Berrios, G.E.; Brook, P.: Visual hallucinations and sensory delusions in the elderly. Br. J. Psychiat. *144:* 662–664 (1985).
16 Berrios, G.E.; Ryley, J.P.; Garvey, T.P.N.: Moffat, D.A.: Psychiatric morbidity in subjects with inner ear disease. Clin. Otolaryngol. *13:* 259–266 (1988).
17 Neugebauer, R.; Susser, M.: Epilepsy. Some epidemiological aspects. Psychol. Med. *9:* 207–215 (1979).
18 Dam, A.M.; Frederiksen, A.F.; Olsen, U.S.; Dam, M.: Late-onset epilepsy: etiologies of seizure, and value of clinical investigation, EEG, and computerized tomography scan. Epilepsia *26:* 227–231 (1985).
19 Eastwood, M.R.; Corbin, S.L.; Reed, M.; Nobbs, H.; Kedward, H.B.: Acquired hearing loss and psychiatric illness. An estimate of prevalence and co-morbidity in a geriatric setting. B. J. Psychiat. *147:* 552–556 (1985).
20 Shulman, A.; Subjective idiopathic tinnitus: a review. J. Lar. *4:* 1–9 (1981).
21 Zulch, K.J.: Brain tumours, their biology and pathology (Springer, New York 1965).
22 Jones, R.D.: Epidemiology of brain tumours in man and their relationship with chemical agents. Food Chem. Toxicol. *24:* 99–103 (1986).
23 Sutherland, G.R.; Florell, R.; Louw, D.; Chi, N.W.; Sima, A.A.: Epidemiology of primary intracranial neoplasms in Manitoba, Canada. Can. J. neurol Sci. *14:* 586–592 (1987).
24 Lovaste, M.G.; Ferrari, G.; Rossi, G.: Epidemiology of primary intracranial neoplasms. Neuroepidemiology *5:* 220–232 (1986).
25 Koehler, K.; Guth, W.; Grimm, G.: First-rank symptoms of schizophrenia in Schneider-oriented German centers. Archs gen. Psychiat. *34:* 810–813 (1977).
26 Bettes, B.A.; Walker, E.: Positive and negative symptoms in psychotic and other psychiatrically disturbed children. J. Child Psychol. Psychiat. *28:* 555–568 (1987).
27 Levy, J.: Lateral differences in the human brain in cognition and behavioural control; in Buser, Rougeul-Buser, Cerebral correlates of conscious experience (North Holland, New York 1978).
28 Waber, D.: Sex differences in cognition: a function of maturation rate? Science *192:* 572–573 (1976).
29 Bryant, W.S.: De la grande importance psychique des affections d'oreilles. Archs int. Lar. Otol. Rhinol. *23:* 85–98 (1907).
30 Berrios, G.E.; Brook, P.: The Charles Bonnet syndrome and the problems of visual perception in the elderly. Age Ageing *11:* 17–23 (1982).
31 Zatorre, R.J.: Musical perception and cerebral function: a critical review. Music Percept. *2:* 196–221 (1984).
32 Gardner, H.; Silverman, J.; Denes, G.; Semenza, C.; Rosenstiel, A.K.: Sensitivity to musical denotation and connotation in organic patients. Cortex *13:* 242–256 (1977).
33 Critchley, M.; Henson, R.A. (eds): Music and the brain. Studies in the neurology of music (Heinemann, London 1977).
34 Clynes, M. (ed): Music, mind, and brain. The neuropsychology of music (Plenum Press, New York 1982).
35 Bazhin, E.F.; Wasserman, L.I.; Tonkonogii, I.M.; Auditory hallucinations and left temporal lobe pathology. Neuropsychologia *13:* 481–487 (1975).
36 Trimble, M.R.: The neurology of schizophrenia. Br. med. Bull. *43:* 587–598 (1987).
37 Malone, G.L.; Leiman, H.I.: Differential diagnosis of palinacousis in a psychiatric patient. Am. J. Psychiat. *140:* 1067–1068 (1983).
38 Jacobs, L., Feldman, M.; Diamond, S.P.: Palinacusis: persistent or recurring auditory sensations. Cortex *9:* 275–282 (1973).

G.E. Berrios
Department of Psychiatry
University of Cambridge
Addenbrooke's Hospital (Level 4)
Hills Road
Cambridge CB2 2QQ (UK)

Psychopathology 1991;24:361–364

0254–4962/91/0246–0361$2.75/0

Visual Pseudohallucinations: Psychotherapy Case Study of a Long-Standing Perceptual Disorder

C.E. Bacon

Department of Psychotherapy, St. James's University Hospital, Leeds, UK

Abstract. The case of a woman with severe neurosis, seen in once weekly psychotherapy over a period of 3 years, illustrates many of the characteristics of pseudohallucinations: their relation to personality, to sensory deprivation and isolation, and to developmental factors. It also suggests that there may be more than one type of pseudohallucinatory experience.

This 30-year-old woman was not considered to be psychotically ill. She had long-standing problems of disassociation, hypochondriasis, panic and depression. Despite this she had the strengths of intelligence, creativity, verbal ability and perceptiveness about herself and others. She was isolated, and unable to realise her abilities in work, recreation, or relationships.

From early childhood she was lonely and felt different from others in not being able to understand human interactions fully. Her birth was difficult following threatened miscarriages. She suffered from mild diplopia, short sight and recurrent ear infections. Her father was depressive and latterly suffered from ill health. Her mother, an anxious woman, was rather brisk and distant. She recalled boredom and loneliness and some persecution from 4 siblings. She developed a vivid imaginative world, being acutely aware of colours and enjoying natural things. She found an ability to hallucinate visually, and from the age of 5 she was able to see bright clouds or sheaves of flowers in her room and angels, each with their own personality, who would teach her about the world. As evoked companions they helped her with perceptual understanding, giving her instructions on how to make sense of the corners of a room, thus enabling her to get an idea of space, depth and the weight of objects. She was often confined by her parents and not allowed to move around and learn by experimentation and exploration. When told to sit still she would imagine she could scratch her arm when it tickled and thus make herself feel comfortable, using tactile hallucination with an ability similar to self-hypnosis.

Physical symptoms included migrainous headaches often associated with numbness of the left side and visual scotoma. There were 'blackouts', but neurological investigations were negative. Psychological testing showed no evidence of organic perceptual disturbance. An EEG showed no epileptic focus. She gradually withdrew from work and friends. When she entered therapy she had multiple neurotic symptoms. She had difficulty leaving the house and was unwilling to allow friends in. She described two forms of abnormal perception: her 'hallucinations' and her 'pictures'. Both were seen (and occasionally heard or felt) in external space but were recognised as different forms of experience. They occurred against a background of symptoms which had changed little over many years: a chronic state of depersonalisation and derealisation; very little experience of emotional or bodily solidity; her body image sense and position sense were unreliable; body sensation was limited to areas in a band round her chest and a patch around her nose and face and areas where she came into contact with furniture. These abnormalities gave her a feeling of falling and of insecurity. She had little appreciation of perspective. She was also hypersensitive to stimuli and considerably distractible: she was able to hear the therapist's wristwatch while it was in her pocket. She found it hard not to focus on an aspect of clothing (a broken button, mud on shoes), exquisite olfactory acuity told her what sandwiches the therapist had had for lunch. Thought content included images of idealised fantasies of bliss or terrifying visions of violence and destruction, both poles being frequently highly sexualised. This internal world dominated intrusively. It was experienced as sterile imagination related to hopes and wishes but not to volition or execution of plans. Dreams were sterotyped, containing similar fantasies to those of her daytime imaginal world. There was vivid experience but no feeling tone. Dreams ended either with hypnopompic experiences of being comforted by an imaginary figure holding her like a baby, or the compulsive need to cut herself or damage herself vaginally.

The first type of hallucinatory experience was almost entirely visual. Described as her 'hallucinations', these experiences were usually unexpected, suddenly breaking into normal experience with compelling intensity. Hallucinated cats came to represent her fear of closeness, rats gnawing at her limbs appeared when she felt oppressed by the views of others, blood flowed from imaginary wounds when she felt persecuted. When these experiences became very real she was very frightened and could do little to handle them but wait until they disappeared. At other times she could control them. She would get rid of bees buzzing in her jersey by picking them out meticulously while at the same time being aware of the unreality. Another form of control was to cognitively add other sensory modalities, tactile imagination being particularly powerful. To allow herself to be cut by the knife, or bitten by the rat, allowed the vision to fade leaving her with the painful or frightening emotion that can then be understood and mastered psychologically.

More difficult to control were pleasant hallucinations. She still had visions of flowers and bright clouds. Once leaves began to sprout from the therapist's ears. They easily faded, however, leaving her disappointed. It was much more difficult to convert them into pleasurable emotions. Sometimes she saw hallucinatory figures, distinguishing them from real perception by the way they failed to move towards her and by the faint light around them which separated them from the environment. When they occurred her eyes moved rapidly to and from and though she could usually be distracted, they were intrusive and difficult to incorporate into dialogue. These were pseudohallucinations rather than true hallucinations. A degree of subjectivity remained. She saw them as 'part of her story', that is, egosyntonic, and although not fully integrated, potentially controllable in a way that the environment is not controllable. They most closely fit Kräupl-Taylor's [1] description of 'perceived pseudo-hallucination'.

Second are her 'pictures', which were also seen and felt to occur in external space but more clearly recognised as a form of imagination and thus they closely resemble 'imaginal pseudo-hallucinations' [1]. They were experienced as related to pictorial memory and as having function and meaning. Their function is cognitive and related to a sense of wishing to understand the world. Their sense of meaning arises from the feeling of purposeful mental activity. They seemed to occur in states such as boredom or loneliness and fill an affective gap. For example, she was erratic about food, at times binging and at others going without food for several days. In this situation she sometimes spontaneously 'pictured' a desired plate of food which was visualised a few feet in front of her. Using this image she could prepare her meal, matching a real plate and real food with the pictures. The degree of control was not an all or none affair however. Sometimes she was unable to evoke hallucinations, at times an incomplete picture was produced or a faint, ghostlike one.

She used a similar mental activity as a means of coping with imagined fears related to people. She found her therapist frightening, and a variety of hallucinatory experiences occurred in therapy. She sees a monster with claws and fangs like a picture projected onto a screen between herself and the therapist. In order to perceive the therapist in a more real light, the hallucination had to be reversed by an active process.

At times, by means of a negative hallucination, the therapist's face could be erased so that she was left with a partially invisible therapist. Another way of experiencing a frightening face or other aspects which caused alarm (such as high heeled shoes) was for them to be projected into another chair in the room. In this way she could sit beside the therapist and talk, without experiencing incapacitating anxiety. It took effort, sometimes as a result of psychotherapeutic work, in which memories and fantasies of other frightening figures were disentangled, to modify and combine the two elements and return a transformed image, less frightening, to her memory.

Despite these abnormalities in visual perception, she relied most strongly on vision and found it difficult to integrate other modalities of perception, smell, touch, and hearing. She described a difficulty in getting a feeling of depth because she could not imagine texture and shape that come from a tactile imagination and had to use a mental effort to do so. There was also an abnormality in visualisation and visual memory. At times she could not switch off or switch on a visual memory, so that she suffered uncomfortable feelings, either of profound loss, or of mania about objects, and was also unable to anticipate previously experienced events. Like many schizoid or autistic people, she could experience her own mental processes in vivid detail, she objectified herself and her imagination and thus deprived herself of a deep sense of subjectivity and the texture of feelings. But this very deficit gave a clear concept of functioning of the perceptual apparatus. Perception is a two-way process, she said 'like radar sending out signals to discover the world'. It entails not only receiving information through the senses but also sending out the information of imagination and memory, projecting and matching what is within to the external world so as to achieve a real sense of connection. This patient illustrates the incapacitating effect of perceptual disturbance in the non-psychotic and the range of phenomena covered by the term pseudohallucination. The case raises questions about the nature of 'normal' and 'abnormal' imagination and its function in relation to memories and to the development of meaningful perception and action.

Reference

Kräuptl-Taylor, F.: On pseudo-hallucinations. Psychol. Med. *11:* 265–271 (1981).

C.E. Bacon
Department of Psychotherapy
St. James's University Hospital
Beckett Street
Leeds LS9 7TF (UK)

Psychopathology 1991;24:365–368

0254–4962/91/0246–0365$2.75/0

Lateralized Anomalous Perceptual Experiences in Schizophrenia

R. Persaud, J. Cutting

Bethlem Royal Hospital, London, UK

Abstract. Four cases of schizophrenia are described, in which subjects reported anomalous perceptual experiences confined to one visual field, in all cases the left visual field. The pattern, content and laterality of such anomalous perceptions point to the presence of right hemisphere dysfunction in schizophrenia. Further evidence to this effect comes from examining the type of anomalous perceptual experiences reported by subjects with focal lesions in either hemisphere. Those with right hemisphere damage but not those with left hemisphere damage report almost identical experiences to those seen in the 4 schizophrenics described here.

Anomalous perceptual experiences, particularly in the visual modality, are frequently reported by schizophrenics, especially at the outset of their first episode [Matussek, 1952; Conrad, 1958; Cutting and Dunne, 1986]. The essence of an anomalous perception is that the object concerned, for example a face, is still recognised as a face, but is perceived in a *distorted* way – crooked, discoloured, etc. The perceptual abnormality contrasts both with an illusion where an object is perceived as entirely different from how it really is and an hallucination when an object is perceived despite its absence in reality. Jaspers [1959] made this distinction clearly and neurologists often refer to the phenomenon of anomalous perceptions as metamorphopsias [Critchley, 1953]. In a neurological context, they are particularly common following parietal lesions. The objects and qualities of the world which form the focus of such anomalous perceptions are very varied, but the most common in schizophrenia are faces and colours [Cutting and Dunne, 1986]. The purpose of this article is to describe a further characteristic, which, to our knowledge, has not been previously reported, namely anomalous perceptual experiences confined to one visual field.

Case Reports

Case 1. A man of 24 was referred to the senior author with a 2-year history of altered perceptual experiences involving his own face and the faces of others, particularly his mother's and his sister's. He had the somatic experience that the left side of his own face had become swollen, and when he looked in the mirror, the same side (left but appearing as the right in the mirror) was darker than the other side. The faces of his mother and sister, and to a lesser extent other people's faces, also looked darker than usual. In the case of his mother, her whole face looked black to begin with, but over the course of a few weeks, this change settled to the right side only.

There was no history of psychiatric disorder in his immediate relatives. He had been outstandingly successful academically, and his symptoms began while a medical student. He had been suspended from his studies when we saw him, because of a previous psychiatrist's report that he was schizophrenic.

At interview he displayed some blunting of affect, used some words to mean something quite different from their dictionary meaning, and had a complex delusional system based on his anomalous perceptual experiences. For example, he believed that his facial change stemmed from the fact that he had once read some pornographic literature and the changes in other people's faces were a physiological consequence of their contact with pornography.

No abnormal neurological signs were detected on clinical examination. A CT scan and EEG were normal. Neuropsychological testing revealed a verbal IQ of 136 and a performance IQ of 108 on the Wechsler Adult Intelligence Scale (WAIS). The only abnormality on more specific tests for lateralized dysfunction emerged in the course of the Rey-Osterrieth test, where his memory of the complex figure was reported as 'haphazard'.

Following a period on neuroleptic treatment he lost all his symptoms, and at 1-year follow-up he is apparently normal. His medical school still refuses to allow him to continue his studies.

Case 2. A man of 21 was admitted to a psychiatric hospital with a 2-year history of social decline. From being a promising art student, and obtaining top marks in his first year at art college, he had deteriorated to a state where he stared into space during classes and was neglecting his self-care.

During his admission he exhibited a range of first rank symptoms of schizophrenia, including third person auditory hallucinations commenting on his behaviour, thought insertion and thought withdrawal.

He also reported anomalous experiences in the visual modality. He declared seeing, out of the corner of his left eye, people's faces as distorted, 'as if they were evil'. When he turned his head to look face on with both eyes, the distortions would disappear, and the faces would look normal again. Houses and windows also appeared distorted if he looked at them in the periphery of his left field of vision, and whole scenes would appear darker and 'unreal'. He said that the distorted faces made people look like 'space aliens'. His mother had held peculiar beliefs about witchcraft for many years, but had not seen a psychiatrist.

Neurological examination was normal, as was a CT scan and an EEG. On the WAIS he had a full scale IQ of 97. His Rey-Osterrieth performance was well below average, with a delayed recall of only 27%. Treatment with neuroleptics eventually produced remission of his symptoms.

Case 3. A man of 20 of Afro-Caribbean origin was admitted to a forensic psychiatric unit following an unprovoked attack on a shopkeeper. He was exhibiting auditory hallucinations, formal thought disorder and thought withdrawal on admission.

He reported that the left side of his face *felt* darker and the same side (i.e. right in mirror) *appeared* darker in the mirror than the other side. He also believed that the acne on the same side looked worse than on the other, although this was not objectively apparent. He was reluctant to allow nurses to escort him on the left side of his body, attaching some sinister significance to this, about which he would not talk. He believed that the medication which he was prescribed only worked on the right side of his brain, whereas the left side was 'just water, not solid'. He had an identical twin who had also been diagnosed as schizophrenic.

Neurological, CT scan and EEG examinations were normal. His verbal IQ on the WAIS was 72, his performance IQ 64. After a course of neuroleptics at therapeutic levels he lost all his symptoms.

Case 4. A man of 38 was admitted to hospital following 2 weeks of distressing changes in the way he saw the world. He remembered them as follows: 'From my flat I can see the aeroplanes on their way to Heathrow Airport. There was something radically wrong with them when I saw them out of my left eye only. They did not look right, although they had the right shape. Also I noticed that, although I knew they were on their way to the airport and must be receding into the distance, to me they looked as if they were getting nearer. It was all very frightening. Also when I looked at a clock I found I could not tell the time, although I could see the clock and the hands perfectly well.' He had said at one time that one side of the clock looked different from the other, but denied this to us. He held delusions about his body and believed that people around him were withdrawing emotions from him.

Neurological examination was normal, as was his CT scan. He would not agree to undergo neuropsychological testing. He refused all medication and discharged himself against medical advice.

Discussion

All 4 cases, with otherwise typical schizophrenic phenomena, experienced lateralized anomalous experiences in the left visual field. Such a phenomenon clearly implicates right hemisphere dysfunction. Despite normal CT scans and EEGs in the 2 patients who complied with neuropsychological testing, there was poor performance on the Rey-Osterrieth test, a good measure of right hemisphere dysfunction [Lezak, 1983]. Although there are reports of delusions about the body having a left-sided preponderance in schizophrenia [Taylor and Fleminger, 1981], there are no reports to our knowledge of the same lateralization for anomalous visual experiences. The significance of the issue lies in suggestions over the last 20 years that schizophrenia is associated with hemisphere imbalance. This was first proposed by Flor-Henry [1969]. He came to the conclusion that left hemipshere dysfunction was the underlying cause. Since then, however, other investigators have proposed different patterns of hemisphere imbalance – left hemisphere overactivity [Gur, 1978], left and right dysfunction in different varieties of schizophrenia [Gruzelier, 1981] and right hemisphere dysfunction alone [Cutting, 1985].

It is our contention that these 4 cases of otherwise typical schizophrenia support the last suggestion. Moreover, examination of case reports of anomalous visual experiences reported by patients who have sustained definite focal damage to one or the other hemisphere gives further support to this proposal. Cutting [1990] has reviewed 26 cases of left-sided (7 cases) or right-sided damage (19 cases) causing anomalous visual perceptions.

In the former group of cases, the anomalous perceptions consisted of major geometrical displacements of things around them. The 'lower half of a vertical line was bent, as if refracted in water' [Best, 1917]. People and objects were 'not distorted but toppled over 45° to the right' [Pichler, 1943]. Landscape seemed 'untidy, piled up, as if blasted by a bomb' [Critchley, 1951]. Furniture seemd 'turned around' [Critchley, 1953]. Or else objects seemed endowed with a special significance – flowers extraordinarily beautiful, the stranger in a park seemed to be a man of great importance [Critchley, 1951].

Patients with right hemisphere lesions, on the other hand, reported a different set of anomalous experiences. The sizes and relative distances of things were particularly affected – 'windows looked excessively small, people looked too small' [van Bogaert, 1934]; 'my husband seemed too big and yet a long way away' [Critchley, 1953]. Of particular interest in relation to the 4 schizophrenics described in this article, several patients reported changes in their experience of movement of objects or distortions confined to the left field of vision. 'Everyone's skull looked flattened on the left (his left field, their right hemiface), and the hair there looked grey and mouldy' [Pichler, 1943]. Stationary objects 'seemed to be moving towards me' [Pichler, 1943]. 'Other people seemed suddenly to move very quickly' [Pichler, 1943]. 'Everything on the left side looked 1½ times as big as that on the right' [Lenz, 1949]. 'Everything on my left side had a disagreeable quality' [Teuber et al., 1960]. 'Half of people's faces in my left field of vision seemed to melt away like clocks in a Dali painting' [Brust and Behrens, 1977].

The last group of reports are quite similar to the experiences of our schizophrenics, and support the notion that right hemisphere dysfunction is involved in this condition.

References

Best, F.: Hemianopsie und Seelenblindheit bei Hirnverletzungen. Archs Ophthal. *93:* 49–150 (1917).

Brust, J.C.M.; Behrens, M.M.: 'Release hallucinations' as the major symptom of posterior artery occlusion: a report of 2 cases. Ann. Neurol. *2:* 432–436 (1977).

Conrad, K.: Die beginnende Schizophrenie (Thieme, Stuttgart 1958).

Critchley, M.: Types of visual perseveration: 'paliopsia' and 'illusory visual spread'. Brain *74:* 267–299 (1951).

Critchley, M.: The parietal lobes (Hafner, New York 1953).

Cutting, J.: The psychology of schizophrenia (Churchill Livingstone, Edinburgh 1985).

Cutting, J.; Dunne, F.: The nature of the abnormal perceptual experiences at the onset of schizophrenia. Psychopathology *19:* 347–352 (1986).

Cutting, J.: The right hemisphere and psychiatry (Oxford University Press, Oxford 1990).

Flor-Henry, P.: Psychosis and temporal lobe epilepsy: a controlled investigation. Epilepsia *10:* 363–395 (1969).

Gruzelier, J.: Hemispheric imbalances masquerading as paranoid and nonparanoid syndromes? Schizophr. Bull. *7:* 662–673 (1981).

Gur, R.E.: Left hemisphere dysfunction and left hemisphere overactivation in schizophrenia. J. abnorm. Psychol. *87:* 226–238 (1978).

Jaspers, K.: General psychopathology; 7th ed. (Springer-Verlag, Berlin 1959).

Lenz, H.: Über zentral bedingte Störungen des Grössensehens. Festschrift zum 70. Geburtstag von O. Pötzl, pp. 315–322 (Universitäts-Verlag Wagner, Innsbruck 1949).

Lezak, M.: Neuropsychological assessment; 2nd ed. (Oxford University Press, New York 1983).

Matussek, P.: Untersuchungen über die Wahnwahrnehmung. Arch. Psychiat. NervKrankh. *189:* 279–318 (1952).

Pichler, E.: Über Störungen des Raum- und Zeiterlebens bei Verletzungen des Hinterhauptlappens. Z. ges. Neurol. Psychiat. *176:* 434–464 (1943).

Taylor, P.; Fleminger, J.J.: The lateralization of symptoms in schizophrenia. Br. J. Med. Psychol. *54:* 59–65 (1981).

Teuber, H.-L.; Battersby, W.S.; Bender, M.B.: Visual field defects after penetrating missile wounds of the brain (Harvard University Press, Cambridge 1960).

Van Bogaert, L.: Sur des changements métriques et formels de l'image visuelle dans les affections cérébrales. J. Belge Neurol. *34:* 717–725 (1934).

R. Persaud, MD
Bethlem Royal Hospital and Maudsley Hospitals
Denmark Hill
Camberwell
London (UK)

Psychopathology 1991;24:369–374

0254–4962/91/0246–0369$2.75/0

An Overview of the Psychopathology of Perception: First Rank Symptoms as a Localizing Sign in Schizophrenia

Andrew Sims

Department of Psychiatry, St. James's University Hospital, Leeds, UK

Abstract. Schneider considered that first rank symptoms always signify schizophrenia. They appear to have in common permeability of the barrier between the individual and his environment, or a loss of ego boundaries. They may be a manifestation of a specific disturbance which may be caused pathologically by a limbic lesion in the dominant hemisphere.

Psychopathology should be accessible to the normal methods of scientific investigation; it should be quantifiable. This was exemplified by a demonstration of how the *perceptual span* can be used as a way to measure abnormality in different types of hysterical disorder (Mace). Psychopathology must also begin with a clear description of the phenomena, as was shown in an account of near-death experiences (Roberts).

The psychopathology of perception above all else concerns the aspect of meaning – the meaning attached to disturbance in perception. So a cognitive account of hallucination demonstrates that an internal event is inferred to be an outside event (Bentall). A schizophrenic patient hears a hallucinatory voice saying about her: 'She is looking for her obituary in the Daily Express . . . she's a stuck up cow'. More important than the voice is its meaning.

The search for meaning becomes a unifying factor in the psychopathology of schizophrenia. Disorders of perception, such as hallucinations and especially auditory hallucinations, and disorder of body image, especially passivity or delusions of control, are then seen to be much closer conceptually. They may both represent disorders of the boundaries of oneself (see below).

Phenomenology and Brain Pathology

It is postulated [McKenna, 1987] that positive symptoms of schizophrenia may be the result of functional dopamine excess and that the features of the condition are determined by the sites at which this neurochemical abnormality occurs. Evidence is as follows: (1) It has been demonstrated that dopamine agonist drugs are able to induce schizophreniform mental states [Randrup and Munkvad, 1967]; (2) effective neuroleptic drugs so far described have always acted as dopamine antagonists [Carlsson and Lindqvist, 1963]; (3) according to one group, it is only the positive symptoms of schizophrenia, that respond to these psychotropic agents [Johnstone et al., 1978]; (4) increased receptor binding of dopamine is found in the brains of both drug-free subjects [Crawley et al., 1986], and also in drug-naive schizophrenic patients [Wong et al., 1986].

The ascending dopamine pathways in the brain form the mesotelencephalic system. This acts in two distinct ways: (1) It has a diffuse modulatory function distinct from the classical model of neurotransmission, and (2) it acts by mediation of the reinforcement effects of brain stimulation. With this mechanism, schizophrenia may be considered to produce progressive damage to the central reward system of the brain. A number of brain structures receive dopaminergic innervations, and an association may be hypothesized involving some of the psychopathological abnormalities of schizophrenic illness. These are summarized in table 1.

Basal ganglia provide the effector system for instrumental learning and performance: there are extensive links with the motor cortex. Dopamine facilitates the passage of information in the striopallidal circuit; that is, its action is *reinforcing*. In 14% of non-geriatric schizophrenic patients never exposed to neuroleptics, tardive-dyskinesia-like symptoms and other motor symptoms with involuntary movements were demonstrated [Crane, 1973].

The ventral striatum controls motor aspects of functions which mediate the animal's arousal by orientation towards and investigation of significant stimuli in the environment. Dopamine excess results in repetitive rhythmic movements. A possible analogue in schizophrenia is the symptom of *parakinesia* consisting of 'fragmentary movements which resemble those of chorea, athetosis and the tics. Although they look like involuntary movements they can always be imitated and are partly reminiscent of expressive and intentional movements' [Fish, 1957].

The septo-hippocampal system compares 'actual' with 'expected' in the animals' environment. Dopamine may be used therefore

Table 1. Sites of mesotelencephalic dopamine innervation [after McKenna, 1987]

Structure	Suggested function	Postulated schizophrenic symptoms
Basal ganglia	instrumental learning and performance	involuntary movements
Ventral striatum	motor aspects of arousal	parakinesia, catatonic mannerism, stereotypy
Septo-hippocampal system	compare actual with expected	delusional meaning and belief
Prefrontal cortex	choice of complex behaviour	formal thought disorder
Dominant hemisphere	verbal function	overinclusiveness, language disorder
Amygdaloid complex	process affective qualities of reinforcing events	bizarre and incongruous mood
Anterior cingulate cortex	vocalisation and auditory decoding	?verbal auditory hallucinations

in this context to label what is 'important, associated with reward'. In schizophrenia the abnormal attribution of significance to neutral events in *delusion* may be evidence of abnormality at this site. Thus the 'specific neuronal machinery for belief' [McKenna, 1987] may be undermined by dopamine excess. Predictions that have not in fact been fulfilled are confirmed in this abnormality as having been matched – there is resonance here with the finding that hallucinations are associated with the attribution of the subject's own speech rather than with perception; the perception is normal but is attributed to outside the self.

The prefrontal cortex has an executive role in the formation, monitoring and revision of behavioural strategies. It gives temporal structure to complex, goal-directed behaviour. The dominant hemisphere is concerned with verbal functions. In schizophrenia, abnormality may be associated with formal thought disorder, loss of goals, language disorder, schizophrenic dysphasia, agrammatism and paragrammatism, neologism, over-inclusiveness and use of stock words and phrases [Sims, 1988].

The amygdaloid complex, which comprises the nuclei of the amygdala, the piriform cortex and stria terminalis, coordinates emotional reactions to perceptual stimuli and processes the affective quality of reinforcing events. Disturbance in schizophrenia may account for bizarre and incongruous mood, and perhaps also for hallucinations. This may link the statement that hallucinations do not fundamentally reveal a defect of perception but much more the way the perceptions are dealt with as messages (Hoffman).

The anterior cingulate cortex is possibly involved in the voluntary initiation of vocalization and auditory decoding by allowing the animal to 'subtract' its own activity from the background of acoustic information: 'If an analogous anatomical arrangement existed in man, if it were devoted to the particular species-specific vocalization of speech, if its 'subtractive' function were damaged by a dopamine excess, might it not be verbal auditory hallucinations that would be the result?' [McKenna, 1987].

Left-sided brain dysfunction is prominent in schizophrenia [Flor-Henry and Gruzelier, 1983]. Positive symptoms of schizophrenia may be associated with dopamine excess and are usually episodic in nature; negative symptoms are more likely to be associated with dopamine deficiency and are in general more prolonged or permanent.

First Rank Symptoms and Schizophrenia

First rank symptoms of schizophrenia were delineated by Schneider in 1939 and are listed in table 2; they were described as an empirical diagnostic list and are all *positive symptoms* [Crow, 1980]. It has been pointed out [Berrios, 1985] that *positive* and *negative symptoms,* as used for epilepsy [Reynolds, 1861; Hughlings Jackson, 1881], implied the mechanism accounting for the symptom as well as its description. Positive

Table 2. First rank symptoms [from Mellor, 1970]

Audible thoughts	Thought withdrawal
Voices arguing	'Made' affect
Voices commenting	'Made' impulse
Somatic passivity	'Made' volition
Thought broadcasting	Delusional percept
Thought insertion	

symptoms in schizophrenia have been considered to indicate the presence of a type 1 schizophrenic syndrome [Wing, 1978], and negative symptoms occur as part of a type 2 syndrome [Crow, 1980]; this contention for schizophrenia therefore also holds implications for the mechanism. Amongst other positive symptoms of schizophrenia, the advantage of using first rank symptoms is that there is fairly general agreement as to definition and usage.

First rank symptoms are regarded as primary symptoms. Schneider [1975] gives six different meanings for the term primary, one of these states: 'From the standpoint of psychopathology primary symptoms are final and irreducible, in the sense in which psychiatrists used to think of "primary" delusions ... anything which is not reducible in psychopathological terms must be organic'. First rank symptoms were described and elegantly demonstrated in the English language literature [Mellor, 1970]. Whether they are pathognomonic of schizophrenia or not has been questioned [Silverstein and Harrow, 1978], and their clinical application has been discussed and extended [Koehler, 1979].

It has been considered that first rank symptoms, as described by Schneider [1957] and Mellor [1970], occur in temporal lobe epilepsy [Trimble, 1986]: 'In patients with temporal lobe epilepsy and psychosis, the latter is likely to be schizophreniform when the dominant hemisphere is primarily affected.' There may be a specific link between first rank symptoms and left-sided brain dysfunction in schizophrenia [Connolly et al., 1983]. There is some evidence for schizophrenia being associated with a lesion in the left limbic area, for example, the temporal pole amygdala. Increased amygdalar dopamine has been found in the left cerebral hemisphere of schizophrenic patients but not in controls. Left-sided cerebral atrophy has been demonstrated in CAT scans, this especially affected limbic structures. It can be postulated that dysfunction arising from the limbic abnormalities in schizophrenia may be particularly associated with the occurrence of first rank symptoms.

First Rank Symptoms

A possible common feature of first rank symptoms is the merging of the usually clear distinction between what is perceived as *self* and *not self*. Schneider [1957] stated that they were not conceived as

> theoretical possibilities, but are intended only for pragmatic diagnostic use ... Some of them can, of course, be grouped together under the concept of 'permeability' of the barrier between the individual and his environment, the so-called 'loss of ego boundaries'. The first rank symptoms which come under the heading of 'ego disturbance' are: thought withdrawal, thought control, thought diffusion, and everything that the patient experiences as 'imposed' on him in the spheres of feeling, drive and volition. Hallucinations of the special senses ... and delusions cannot be brought within this formula without modifying the concept.

However work on the treatment of hallucinations by focussing (Slade) could be considered to support the notion that hallucinations of the special senses, that is auditory hallucinations of first rank, could also be seen within the concept of permeability of the barrier between self and not self. Focussing involves directing attention to the hallucinations thereby bypassing the central monitor and thus ensuring that the patient reattributes what he previously considered to be 'not self', to 'self'.

This disturbance can be seen as an underlying component of both delusional percept and auditory hallucinations as they occur in schizophrenia. For an instance of delusional percept a man asks for bacon for his breakfast and is served a sausage. Immediately it arrives on the plate, he knows with absolute certainty that other people regard him as homosexual. Thus his perception of an object and an event that is actually outside himself and entirely neutral towards himself, is perceived accurately but interpreted as something with great personal meaning involving his own self – in effect, an invasion of the boundaries of self. One interpretation of the description of hallucinations (Cutting) is that the individual attaches delusional mood, ideas of self-reference and personal meaning, intrinsic characteristics of the self, to percepts that are in fact arising outside the self.

Therefore all first rank symptoms may imply loss of ego boundaries. The patient, of course, is not aware of the nature of this, but describes the problem as 'other people are doing things to me, events take place outside myself'. It is the external observer or interviewer who finds the disturbance in the boundaries of the patient's self rather than the patient.

The experience of auditory comments made about himself in the third person singular demonstrates extreme confusion of the boundaries of self: a healthy person or a neurotically disturbed person will regularly think of himself and perhaps even speak about himself in the first person. At times of stress such a person may well address himself silently or aloud in the second person. However, it is never part of our normal experience to think or speak of ourselves in the third person. It demonstrates considerable disruption of the cohesiveness of self-concept so to do.

Hearing one's own thoughts aloud implies locating the innermost core experiences, one's own thought, in outer space; again this demonstrates a massive disturbance in the boundaries of self. Voices arguing or discussing with each other may imply the location of a conflict that is actually private, inside the self as something external to self. The innermost cisterns of self-knowledge, and self-doubt, have become permeable and are leaking.

With passivity experiences functions ascribed to 'not self' arise inside the self. The patient describing passivity of impulse claims 'my arm lifted itself against my will and hit the other person without my intending to do it. It was made to do that'. First rank symptoms therefore can be seen specifically to indicate disturbance in the boundaries of self. Since this is such an important part of the diagnosis of schizophrenia, perhaps the neuropathological link is a lesion in the limbic system of the dominant hemisphere.

References

Berrios, G.E.: Positive and negative symptoms and Jackson: a conceptual history. Archs gen. Psychiat. *42:* 95–97 (1985).

Carlsson, A.; Lindqvist, M.: Effect of chlorpromazine and haloperidol on formation of 3-methoxytyramine and normetanephrine in mouse brain. Acta pharmac. tox. *20:* 140–144 (1963).

Connolly, J.F.; Gruzelier, J.H.; Manchanda, R.: Electrocortical and perceptual asymmetries in schizophrenia; in Flor-Henry, Gruzelier, Laterality and psychopathology (Elsevier, Amsterdam 1983).

Crane, G.E.: Persistent dyskinesia. Br. J. Psychiat. *122:* 395–405 (1973).

Crawley, J.C.W.; Crow, T.J.; Johnstone, E.C.; Oldland, S.R.D.; Owen, F., et al.: Dopamine D2

receptors in schizophrenia studied in vivo. Lancet *ii:* 224–225 (1986).
Crow, T.J.: Positive and negative schizophrenic symptoms and the role of dopamine. Br. J. Psychiat. *137:* 383–396 (1980).
Fish, F.J.: The classification of schizophrenia: the views of Kliest and his co-authors. J. ment. Sci. *103:* 443–463 (1957).
Flor-Henry, P.; Gruzelier, J.: Laterality and psychopathology (Elsevier, Amsterdam 1983).
Jackson, H.J.: Remarks on the dissolution of the nervous system as exemplified by certain postepileptic conditions (1881); in Taylor, Selected writings of Hughlings Jackson (Staples, London 1958).
Johnstone, E.C.; Crow, T.J.; Frith, C.D.; Carney, M.W.L.; Price, J.S.: Mechanisms of the antipsychotic effect in the treatment of acute schizophrenia. Lancet *i:* 848–851 (1978).
Koehler, K.: First rank symptoms of schizophrenia: questions concerning clinical boundaries. Br. J. Psychiat. *134:* 236–248 (1979).
McKenna, P.J.: Pathology, phenomenology and the dopamine hypothesis of schizophrenia. Br. J. Psychiat. *151:* 288–301 (1987).
Mellor, C.S.: First-rank symptoms of schizophrenia. Br. J. Psychiat. *117:* 15–23 (1970).
Randrup, A.; Munkvad, I.: Stereotyped activities produced by amphetamine in several animal species and man. Psychopharmacologia *11:* 300–310 (1967).
Reynolds, J.R.: Epilepsy: its symptoms, treatment and relations to other chronic convulsive diseases (Churchill, London 1861).
Schneider, K.: Psychischer Befund und psychiatrische Diagnose; English transl. from 5th ed. Clinical Psychopathology 1959 (Grune & Stratton, New York 1939).
Schneider, K.: Primary and secondary symptoms in schizophrenia. Fortschr. Neurol. Psychiat. *25:* 487–490 (1957); transl. H. Marshall in Hirsch, Shepherd, Themes and variations in European psychiatry: an anthology (University Press of Virgina, Charlottesville 1974).
Silverstein, M.L.; Harrow, M.: First rank symptoms in post-acute schizophrenia: a follow-up study. Am. J. Psychiat. *135:* 1481–1486 (1978).
Sims, A.C.P.: Symptoms in the mind (Baillière Tindall, London 1988).
Trimble, M.R.: Positive and negative symptoms in psychiatry. Br. J. Psychiat. *148:* 587–589 (1986).
Wing, J.K.: Clinical concepts of schizophrenia; in Wing, Schizophrenia: towards a new synthesis (Academic Press, London 1978).
Wong, D.F.; Wagner, H.N.; Tune, L.E.; et al.: Positron emission tomography reveals elevated D2 dopamine receptors in drug-naive schizophrenics. Science *234:* 1558–1563 (1986).

Professor A.C.P. Sims, MA., MD., FRCPsych.
Department of Psychiatry
St. James's University Hospital
Leeds LS9 7TF (UK)

Psychopathology 1991;24:375–380

0254–4962/91/0246–0375$2.75/0

Tilt Aftereffect Reveals Early Visual Processing Deficits in Parkinson's Disease and in Chronic Schizophrenic Patients on Depot Neuroleptic

J.E. Calvert[a], *J.P. Harris*[a], *O.T. Phillipson*[b]

[a]Perceptual Systems Research Centre, Department of Psychology, and [b]Department of Anatomy, University of Bristol, UK

Abstract. Previous studies suggest that the tilt aftereffect (TAE) may be used to indicate the site of dopaminergic abnormalities in the human visual system. In this study we investigated the TAE in patients with Parkinson's disease, and in chronic schizophrenic patients receiving depot injections of neuroleptic. The results suggest that the retina may be abnormal in both groups of patients, and that schizophrenic patients may also have cortical changes. The results are discussed in terms of the clinical implications of these visual changes.

Introduction

Evidence is accumulating from both animal [Iuvone et al., 1978; Godley et al., 1985; Jensen and Daw, 1986] and human [Domenici et al., 1985; Bodis-Wollner et al., 1982] studies that dopamine (DA) may be important in early visual processing [for reviews, see Ehinger, 1983; Bodis-Wollner and Piccolino, 1988]. In recent reports [Calvert et al., 1987, 1990; Harris and Calvert, 1989] we have shown that the tilt aftereffect may be a suitable psychophysical tool for providing clues about the location of abnormalities in DA function in the human visual system.

The tilt aftereffect (TAE) is the apparent change in orientation induced in a line or grating following inspection of a line or grating of similar (but not identical) orientation. It almost certainly involves cortical mechanisms, since orientation-selective cells are not found earlier in the visual system. However, since changes in the contrast of the adapting and test stimuli are important in regulating the size of the TAE [Harris and Calvert, 1989], retinal mechanisms may also be involved, since retina is an important site of contrast coding. We have found [Harris and Calvert, 1989] that the size of the TAE depends (among other things) upon both the duration of the test stimulus (declining as the stimulus is prolonged, as shown by Wolfe, 1984), and upon the contrast of the adapting and test stimuli (at short test durations, low contrast stimuli give smaller TAEs than high contrast stimuli, while at long test durations the reverse is true). Thus at short test durations the size of the TAE may reflect the amount of excitation present in the retinal inputs to cortical channels, while at long test durations the size of the TAE may reflect adaptation in the cortical neurones themselves [see Harris and Calvert, 1989, for more details]. We have also shown [Calvert et al., 1990] that the administration of *L*-dopa to normal volunteers has effects which are entirely consistent with the suspected actions of DA in retina (i.e. to regulate light adaptation, and hence contrast perception) [Ehinger, 1983]; and further, that (if the above ideas are correct) DA may act at a cortical level to affect the adaptation of orientation channels (consistent with known projections from the ventral tegmentum to cortex [Phillipson et al., 1987]).

In an attempt to understand the role of DA in visual abnormalities, we have studied the TAE in both parkinsonian (PD) patients, and in chronic schizophrenic patients receiving long-term depot neuroleptic. The TAE may allow more precise identification of the nature and site(s) of the visual abnormalities already reported in such patients [Bodis-Wollner and Piccolino, 1988; Harris et al., 1990].

Methods

Subjects

Two separate groups of patients + controls were tested, as follows: (a) 5 PD patients, mean age 64.6 years, all stabilised on dopaminergic medication, together with 5 age- and sex-matched controls; (b) 8 patients with a long-term diagnosis of schizophrenia, mean age 44.4 years, receiving regular injections of depot neuroleptic, tested 1 day before and 2 days after their injection, together with 8 age- and sex-matched controls.

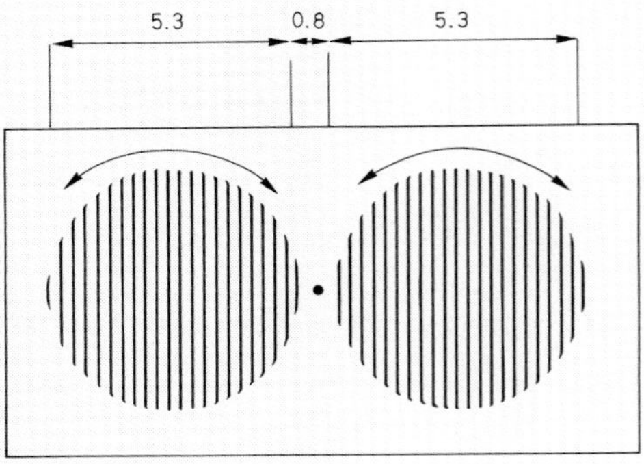

Fig. 1. Schematic representation of the tachistoscopically presented stimuli for measuring the TAE. The subject fixated a central LED between two circular areas of grating. A double interleaved staircase procedure was used to find the point of subjective parallel. During adaptation, each test presentation was preceded by an adapting presentation of 300 ms, in which the tops of the gratings pointed away from each other, each at an angle of 12.5° from the previously measured point of subjective parallel. Dimensions are in degrees of visual angle. See text for more detail.

Materials and Apparatus

A schematic representation of the stimuli is shown in figure 1. These were gratings of either 2 or 10 cycles/degree, whose Michelson contrast was about 0.8, and which could be rotated together about their centres in a symmetrical, mirror-image fashion. These were presented in a tachistosope under computer control at a mean luminance of about 140 cd/m^2, as described below.

Procedure

A randomly interleaved double staircase method was used, in which the computer presented the stimuli, at a predetermined orientation and duration, and the subject was asked to decide whether the tops of the gratings were pointing 'in' or 'out'. In order to induce a TAE, the test gratings were preceded by a set of inducing gratings each oriented 12.5° from vertical in opposite directions. The setting at which the sub-

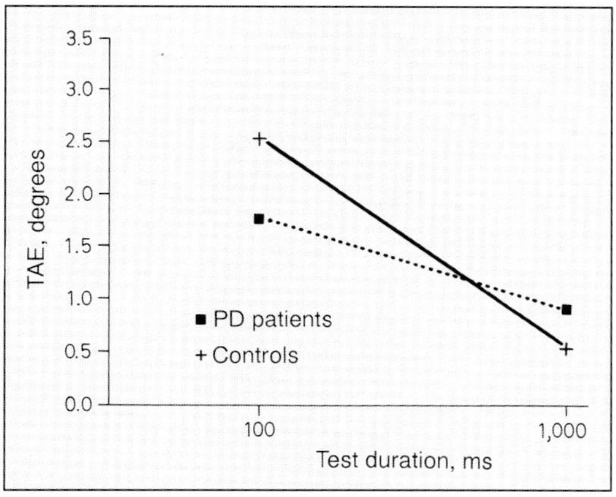

Fig. 2. TAEs produced by 5 patients with PD, and 5 age- and sex-matched controls, using adapting durations of 300 ms, and test durations of either 100 or 1,000 ms, and stimuli of 10 cycles/degree.

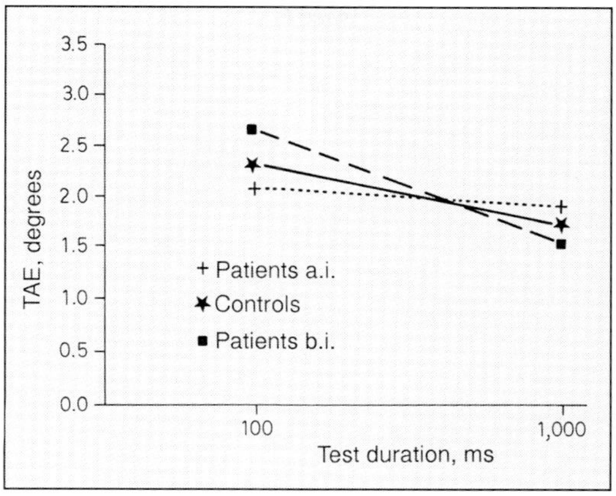

Fig. 3. TAEs produced by 8 patients receiving depot neuroleptic, both before (b.i.) and after (a.i.) their depot injection, and 8 age- and sex-matched controls, using adapting durations of 300 ms, followed by test durations of either 100 or 1,000 ms and stimuli of 10 cycles/degree.

ject judged the gratings to be parallel under these conditions was compared with a control setting made when no inducing gratings were present, and the TAE computed as the difference in apparent parallel between these two conditions. The duration of the inducing gratings was 300 ms, that of the test gratings either 100 or 1,000 ms in any one trial, and the interval between the two was 500 ms [fuller details of this method are given in Harris and Calvert, 1989].

Results

Test Stimuli of 10 Cycles/Degree. The results for the PD patients are shown in figure 2. ANOVA indicates a significant interaction ($p < 0.01$) between subject groups and test duration, and a post hoc Newman-Keuls test demonstrates significant differences between patients and controls at both test durations.

The results for the schizophrenic patients are shown in figure 3. Again, ANOVA indicates a significant interaction between subject groups and test duration ($p < 0.05$), and post hoc Newman–Keuls tests indicate significant differences between patients before and after injection, and between patients before injection and controls at a test duration of 100 ms. At a test duration of 1,000 ms the difference between patients before and after injection approaches significance (critical gap 3.52, actual gap 3.42, for $p < 0.05$).

Test Stimuli of 2 Cycles/Degree. The results for the PD patients are shown in figure 4. ANOVA confirms that patients did not differ significantly from controls. The results for the patients on depot neuroleptic are shown in figure 5. ANOVA reveals a significant interaction between subject groups and test duration, and the Newman-Keuls test indicates significant differences between patients before and after injection, and between patients before injection and controls at 1,000 ms.

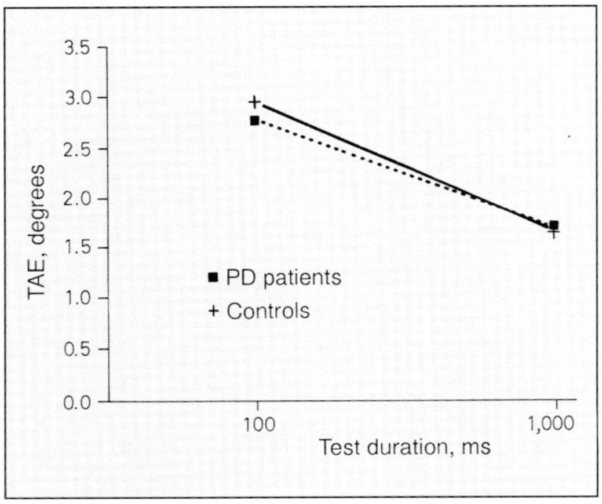

Fig. 4. TAEs produced by 5 patients with PD, and 5 age- and sex-matched controls, using adapting durations of 300 ms, and test durations of either 100 or 1,000 ms, and stimuli of 2 cycles/degree.

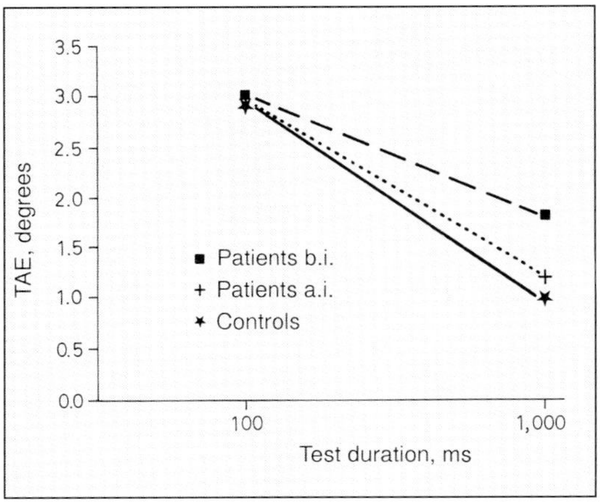

Fig. 5. TAEs produced by 8 patients receiving depot neuroleptic, both before (b.i.) and after (a.i.) their depot injection, and 8 age- and sex-matched control subjects, using adapting durations of 300 ms, followed by test durations of either 100 or 1,000 ms, and stimuli of 2 cycles/degree.

Discussion

With the finer (10 cycles/degree) gratings, PD patients produced results which were opposite to those found when *L*-dopa is given to normal subjects [Calvert et al., 1990], and similar to those seen when the actual contrast of the stimulus is decreased [Harris and Calvert, 1989]. Schizophrenic patients, on the other hand, produce results mimicking an increase in stimulus contrast, and similar to the effects of *L*-dopa, before their injection of neuroleptic (when blood levels of the drug are presumably low). After their injection (when blood levels rise), their results are similar to those of the PD patients. These findings suggest (though of course do not prove) that DA may be acting in the retina to affect contrast perception, which then secondarily affects the excitation of cortical orientation channels, and are consistent with the finding of Domenici et al. [1985] that dopaminergic drugs improve human contrast sensitivity for higher spatial frequencies.

With the coarser (2 cycles/degree) gratings, PD patients showed no significant differences from control subjects. If, as suggested, DA acts to regulate the state of light adaptation, and thus contrast coding, in the retina, the subjective contrast of these relatively low spatial fequencies would be less affected by changes in DA function, so that contrast-related changes might not be expected under these conditions. However, the schizophrenic patients (while, like the PD patients, showing no contrast-related changes at short test durations), do, before their injection, produce larger TAEs at long test durations than controls. Contrast-related effects cannot explain these changes, but they are consistent with our earlier suggestions [Calvert et al., 1990] that DA may affect the neural adaption of orientation channels. (The adaptation to contrast of orientation-selective neurones has been shown to be a cortical phenomenon [Ohzawa et al., 1985].) These results therefore indicate a cortical abnormality in schizophrenia.

We therefore suggest that retinal abnormalities are present in both schizophrenia and in PD, which would act to increase (schizophrenia) or reduce (PD) the subjective perception of contrast at high spatial frequencies. This could explain some of the reports in the literature that schizophrenic patients complain of things appearing too bright [Chapman, 1966; Phillipson and Harris, 1985], or that they are easily distractable. PD patients have been shown to suffer from impaired spatial contrast sensitivity [Kupersmith et al., 1982; Regan and Neima, 1984; Bodis-Wollner, 1988], temporal integration [Harris et al., 1985], and visual neglect [Villardita et al., 1983].

The clinical implications of cortical changes in early visual processing mechanisms, as we suggest may be present in schizophrenia, are not obvious. It has been suggested [Greenlee and Heitger, 1988] that the function of cortical adaptation is to shift the linear region of the contrast response function. If this process were affected, it is possible that ability to discriminate between adjacent contrasts above threshold could be impaired.

Acknowledgements

We thank the Parkinson's Disease Society (J.P.H.) and the Lord Dowding Fund (J.E.C.) for support; Ian Low and Tony Makepeace for technical help; the Bristol Branch of the Parkinson's Disease Society kindly assisted with recruiting members; Dr. I. Babiker and the staff of Glenside Hospital, and the staff of the Industrial Therapy Organisation (Bristol), helped with recruiting patients on depot neuroleptic.

References

Bodis-Wollner, I.: Altered spatio-temporal contrast sensitivity in Parkinson's disease and MPTP-treated monkeys; in Bodis-Wollner, Piccolino (eds): Dopaminergic mechanisms in vision, pp. 205–220 (Liss, New York 1988).

Bodis-Wollner, I.; Piccolino, M. (eds): Dopaminergic mechanisms in vision (Liss, New York 1988).

Bodis-Wollner, I.; Yahr, M.D.; Mylin, L.H.; Thornton, J.: Dopaminergic deficiency and delayed visual evoked potentials in humans. Ann. Neurol. *11:* 478–483 (1982).

Calvert, J.E.; Harris, J.P.; Phillipson, O.T.: Effects of L-dopa on the tilt aftereffect with differing stimulus contrast and test duration. J. Physiol. *384:* 77P (1987).

Calvert, J.E.; Harris, J.P.; Phillipson, O.T.: Effects of L-dopa on the tilt aftereffect with differing stimulus contrast and test duration: implications for schizophrenia and Parkinson's disease. Clin. Vis. Sci. *5:* 87–90 (1990).

Chapman, J.: The early symptoms of schizophrenia. Br. J. Psychiat. *112:* 225–251 (1966).

Domenici, L.; Trimarchi, C.; Piccolino, M.; Fiorentino, A.; Maffei, L.: Dopaminergic drugs improve human visual contrast sensitivity. Human Neurobiol. *4:* 195–197 (1985).

Ehinger, B.: Functional role of dopamine in the retina; in Osbourne, Chader, Progress in Retinal Research, vol. 2 (1983).

Greenlee, M.W.; Heitger, F.: The functional role of contrast adaptation. Vision Res. *28:* 791–797 (1988).

Godley, B.F.; Flaherty, A.W.; Wurtman, R.J.: The effect of light on retinal dopamine in the rat. Ann. N.Y. Acad. Sci. *453:* 383–384 (1985).

Harris, J.P.; Calvert, J.E.: Contrast, spatial frequency and duration effects on the tilt aftereffect: implications for underlying mechanisms. Vision Res. *29:* 129–135 (1989).

Harris, J.P.; Calvert, J.E.; Leendertz, J.A.; Phillipson, O.T.: The influence of dopamine on spatial vision. Eye *4:* 806–812 (1990).

Iuvone, P.M.; Galli, C.L.; Garrison-Gund, C.K.; Neff, N.H.: Light stimulates tyrosine hydroxylase activity and dopamine synthesis in retinal amacrine neurones. Science *202:* 901 (1978).

Jensen, R.J.; Daw, N.W.: Effects of dopamine and its

agonists and antagonists on the receptive field properties of ganglion cells in the rabbit retina. Neuroscience *17:* 837–855 (1986).

Kupersmith, M.J.; Shaken, E.; Siegel, I.; Lieberman, A.: Visual system abnormalities in patients with Parkinson's disease. Arch Neurol. *39:* 284–286 (1982).

Ohzawa, I.; Sclar, G.; Freeman, R.D.: Contrast gain control in the cat's visual system. J. Neurophysiol. *54:* 651–667 (1985).

Phillipson, O.T.; Kilpatrick, I.C.; Jones, M.W.: Dopaminergic innervation of the primary visual cortex in the rat, and some correlations with human cortex. Brain Res. Bull. *18:* 621–633 (1987).

Phillipson, O.T.; Harris, J.P.: Perceptual changes in schizophrenia: a questionnaire survey. Psychol. Med. *5:* 859–866 (1985).

Regan, D.; Neima, D.: Low contrast letter charts in early diabetic retinopathy, ocular hypertension, glaucoma, and Parkinson's disease. Br. J. Ophthal. *68:* 885–889 (1984).

Villardita, C.; Smirni, P.; Zappala, G.: Visual neglect in Parkinson's disease. Archs Neurol. *40:* 737–739 (1983).

Wolfe, J.M.: Short test flashes produce large tilt aftereffects. Vision Res. *24:* 1959–1964 (1984).

J.E. Calvert
Perceptual Systems Research Centre
University of Bristol
Department of Psychology
8 Woodland Road
Bristol BS8 ITN (UK)

Original Papers

Psychopathology 1991;24:381–387

0254–4962/91/0246–0381$2.75/0

Psychiatric and Somatic Hospitalisations of Different Diagnostic Groups: A Long-Term Follow-Up Study

P. Vetter[a], *O. Köller*[b]

Departments of [a]Psychiatry and [b]Psychology, University of Kiel, FRG

Abstract. Out of 328 cases with different diagnoses, including those without pathological findings at follow-up, the frequency and duration of in-patient treatment in psychiatric and somatic institutions was observed over an average 14-year period. Schizophrenics were more frequently and longer in psychiatric institutions, but they were less frequently and for shorter periods in somatic care compared with all other diagnostic groups. Patients suffering from affective psychosis had comparatively long psychiatric and somatic periods of hospitalisation. Dependents were hospitalised more frequently and longer for psychiatric rather than for medical reasons in somatic institutions. The total psychiatric in-patient treatment time was distinctly shorter for neurotic disorders compared with schizophrenic psychosis or affective psychosis cases.

Introduction

To date there has been a lack of long-term follow-up studies on patients with a broad spectrum of different diagnoses [1–7]. Up to now, it has been attempted to obtain study samples that were as homogenic as possible by applying different criteria for exclusion. The aim of this study was to investigate the course of a population that was not bound by narrow nosological classifications or other criteria. To establish this, the question considered was in what way groups of psychiatric disorders differed in number and duration of hospitalisation in the follow-up period. We hypothesized more frequent hospitalisations and longer periods of in-patient treatment in psychiatric institutions for patients suffering from schizophrenic and affective psychosis compared with patients suffering from neurotic disorders (including personality disorders, acute reactions to stress and adjustment disorders). Compared with other diagnostic groups we hypothesized longer in-patient treatment for medical reasons as being due to underlying physical disorders, respectively, noncompliance on the part of patients with an organic mental disorder, dependence as well as nondependent abuse of alcohol [8]. Finally we hypothesized that patients suffering from neurotic disorders were hospitalised more frequently and longer in somatic institutions for psychiatric reasons than other diagnostic groups due, on the one hand, to a higher rate of attempted suicide [9] and due, on the other hand, to frequently occurring functional disorders.

Material and Methods

The study was based on all hospitalised patients (n= 1,114) admitted to the Psychiatric University Clinic in Kiel from January 1 to December 31 1972. The classification of the index diagnoses into their respective diagnosis groups was based on the ICD-9 [10]. All patients who were index-diagnosed as cases of dependence or nondependent abuse of alcohol and drugs (ICD:303, ICD:304, ICD:305), with specific nonpsychotic mental disorders following organic brain damage (ICD:310), as well as those diagnosed with an organic psychotic condition (ICD:290–294), were excluded from the study. 572 patients fulfilled the required criteria. They were classified according to other (nonorganic) psychoses groups (ICD:295–299); neurotic disorders (ICD:300); personality disorders (ICD:301); other nonpsychotic mental disorders (ICD:302, ICD:306–309, ICD:313, ICD:316) and mental retardation (ICD:317, ICD:318).

The index diagnosis of an endogenous psychosis (n = 4) was included in the diagnostic group of schizophrenic psychoses because the initial description and development of the psychopathological clinical picture clearly corresponded to Bleuler's [11] criteria of schizophrenia. The index diagnoses of a physiological malfunction arising from mental factors (n = 6), and special symptoms or syndromes not elsewhere classified (n = 2) were included in the diagnostic group of neurotic disorders, because they were based on a neurotic disorder. The diagnosis group of psychogenic reactions was composed of acute reactions to stress (ICD:308) and adjustment reactions (ICD:309).

Even though a wide spectrum of diagnoses was included, it still was not possible to define several population groups according to certain diagnostic criteria without obtaining a remaining group with heterogenic diagnoses. This group consisted of the following index diagnoses: paranoid psychosis (n = 8; ICD:297.0); involutional paranoid state (n = 1; ICD:297.2); nonorganic psychosis, excitative type (n= 1; ICD:298.1); acute paranoid reaction (n = 1; ICD:298.3); autism (n = 1; ICD:299.0); sexual deviation (n = 1; ICD:302.2); anorexia nervosa (n = 1; ICD:307.1); puberty crisis (n = 3; ICD:313.3); ulcerative colitis (n = 2; ICD:316); mental retardation (n = 5; ICD:317/318) and tactile hallucinosis ('Dermatozoenwahn'; n = 1).

For administrative reasons, the sample of this study consisted of 436 patients. In 29 cases a follow-up was not possible, because the patients could not be located or refused to participate. 79 patients had died. Therefore only 328 patients could be followed up (82% personally, 14% in the form of a telephone interview and 4% by means of secondary sources). Data was collected from June 1985 to August 1988. The mean follow-up period was 14.0 years. Data concerning all psychiatric and somatic hospitalisations in the follow-up period was not only collected in our university hospitals and clinics but also elsewhere. It was only possible to document 98% of the psychiatric and 95% of the somatic hospitalisations. The collection, interviewing and diagnostic classifying of the data was carried out by one of the authors. This approach is recommended by Kringlen [12].

The follow-up diagnoses were based on the ICD-9. All accessible material from hospital records, family doctors, relatives, etc. was taken into consideration. The groups which were formed at the time of the follow-up are shown in the tables. The diagnostic group of organic mental disorders was first included at follow-up. All cases ranging from a psycho-organic syndrome to a dementia without aetiological differentiation were then included when these illnesses were predominant (ICD:290; ICD:291.1; ICD:291.2; ICD:294).

The diagnostic group of dependents was also initially included at follow-up. This group comprised all cases in which the observed symptomatology at index hospitalisation had been replaced at follow-up by symptoms of alcohol and/or drug dependence (ICD:303, ICD:304). The matching group without pathological findings comprised all patients who did not show or reveal any symptoms of clinical value and were found to be psychopathologically negative at follow-up. No indications of a residual state [13] were to be found. These patients were complaint- and symptom-free for at least a year before being interviewed at follow-up. After an average 14-year period, changes in diagnosis are hardly to be expected. The statistical evaluation was, therefore, based solely on the diagnosis made at follow-up, respectively, it was based on the diagnostic groups which were formed from the material [see also 14, 15].

Results

The age and sex distributions of the diagnostic groups are given in table 1. The study of the psychiatric hospitalisation frequencies (table 1) revealed significant mean differences among the groups. Schizophrenics were the most frequently hospitalised with an average of 6.5 hospitalisations during the follow-up period. Cases diagnosed as psychogenic reaction were hospitalised the least and had a mean of 0.5 hospitalisations.

The results of the analysis concerning the total and relative duration in a psychiatric clinic (length of hospitalisation per admission) were analogous to this. Schizophrenics

Table 1. Socio-demographic variables and psychiatric hospitalisations (PH) concerning diagnostic groups

		n	Sex		Age when first hospitalised	Age at index hospitalisation	Total frequency of PH	Total duration of PH weeks	Relative duration of PH weeks
			M	F					
1	Schizophrenic psychosis	54	27	27	27.19[2,3,5,7–9] (8.89)	30.24[2,5,8] (8.94)	6.50[3–6,8,9] (8.63)	119.70[3–9] (176.91)	47.23[3–9] (148.13)
2	Affective psychosis	14	7	7	36.14[1,8] (10.48)	39.33[1,3,8,9] (11.71)	3.36[3–6,8,9] (3.86)	74.55[3–5] (183.35)	9.84[3–5,7,8] (13.01)
3	Neurotic disorder	83	33	50	33.94[1,5,8] (13.12)	34.26[2,5,8] (13.11)	1.42[1,2,7,9] (4.17)	14.51[1,2,4,5] (37.40)	4.96[1,2,9] (11.65)
4	Personality disorder	25	17	8	33.17[5,8] (14.72)	34.80[5,8] (15.10)	1.20[1,2,9] (1.85)	5.27[1–3] (8.02)	1.97[1,2,9] (2.58)
5	Psychogenic reaction	6	2	4	43.95[1,3,4] (13.23)	45.33[1,3,4,6–9] (10.56)	0.50[1,2,7] (1.22)	2.90[1–3] (7.10)	0.97[1,2] (2.37)
6	Heterogenous diagnoses	7h	3	4	30.89[8] (14.14)	33.14[5,8] (9.56)	1.00[1,2] (1.41)	12.37[1] (17.29)	8.36[1] (16.26)
7	Dependence	17	9	8	35.34[1,8] (13.06)	35.80[5,8] (13.01)	4.65[1,3,5,9] (9.31)	17.71[1,9] (39.48)	1.79[1,2,9] (1.89)
8	Organic mental disorders	17	11	6	50.24[1–4,6,7,9] (14.01)	55.59[1–7,9] (12.51)	1.71[1,2,9] (2.71)	30.36[1,9] (74.38)	4.63[1,2] (9.39)
9	Symptom- and complaint-free	105	41	64	33.83[1,5,8] (12.69)	34.31[2,5,8] (13.41)	0.57[1–4,7,8] (1.51)	6.91[1–4,7,8] (30.73)	2.17[1–4,7,8] (6.08)
	Significance		NS		*	*	*	*	*

NS: Non-significant differences; * Significant differences beyond the 1 % level.

Group differences over all diagnostic groups were tested using the χ^2 test for association (for the variable sex) and the Kruskal-Wallis analysis of variance by ranks. The superscript numbers indicate significant differences from the means of other diagnostic groups (Mann-Whitney test, $p < 0.05$).

had, on average, the longest of the psychiatric total hospitalisation time, and they were also hospitalised the longest per admission. Cases diagnosed as psychogenic reaction had the shortest hospitalisation period in both variables. Next to the schizophrenics, cases classified as affective psychosis also had a comparatively long psychiatric total hospitalisation period. Table 2 presents the frequency and duration of all somatic hospital-

Table 2. Frequency and duration of all somatic hospitalisations (SH) including psychiatric-like hospitalisations in somatic institutions (means and standard deviations)

	n	Total frequency of SH	Total duration of SH weeks	Frequency of SH[a] weeks	Total duration of SH[a] weeks	Ratio[b]
1 Schizophrenic psychosis	54	0.56[2,3,5,7–9] (1.57)	1.60[2,3,5,7–9] (4.69)	0.24[3,7] (1.20)	0.42[3,7] (2.09)	0.22 (0.42)
2 Affective psychosis	14	1.13[1,4] (0.99)	3.47[1,4,9] (4.22)	0.20[4,7] (0.56)	0.20[4,7] (0.56)	0.20 (0.42)
3 Neurotic disorder	83	1.49[1,4] (3.86)	3.55[1] (9.47)	0.73[1,4,7] (3.72)	1.64[1,4,7] (8.13)	0.24 (0.40)
4 Personality disorder	25	0.68[2,3,5,7,8] (1.35)	2.60[2,5,7] (6.27)	0.00[2,3,7] (0.00)	0.00[2,3,7,8] (0.00)	0.00 (0.00)
5 Psychogenic reaction	6	1.83[1,4] (2.14)	5.00[1,4] (5.72)	0.00[7] (0.00)	0.00[7] (0.00)	0.00 (0.00)
6 Heterogenous diagnoses	7	1.57 (2.15)	4.29 (8.01)	0.00[7] (0.00)	0.00[7] (0.00)	0.00 (0.00)
7 Dependence	17	1.40[1,4,9] (1.32)	2.60[1,4,9] (2.41)	0.80[1–6,8,9] (1.32)	1.53[1–6,8,9] (2.29)	0.58 (0.50)
8 Organic mental disorders	17	1.47[1,4] (1.97)	3.53[1] (4.87)	0.29[7] (0.85)	0.88[7] (2.64)	0.15 (0.31)
9 Symptom- and complaint-free	105	0.73[1,2,7] (1.07)	1.90[1,2,7] (3.84)	0.21[5,7] (0.73)	0.57[5,7] (3.03)	0.20 (0.37)
Significance		*	*	*	*	NS

NS: Non-significant differences; * Significant differences beyond the 1 % level.

Group differences over all diagnostic groups were tested using the Kruskal-Wallis analysis of variance by ranks. The superscript numbers indicate significant differences from the mean of other diagnostic groups (Mann-Whitney test, $p < 0.05$).

[a] Due to injury/poisoning or functional disorders.

[b] Ratio of hospitalisation duration due to injury/poisoning or functional disorders to total hospitalisation duration in somatic institutions.

isations. All psychiatric-related treatments that took place in somatic hospitals are specified here. Significant differences concerning the total number and duration were revealed among the groups. Compared with cases of all other diagnostic groups, including the group without pathological findings, schizophrenics were treated least frequently and for the shortest time in somatic institutions during the follow-up period. Apart from the small case groups diagnosed as either psychogenic reactions or heterogenic diagnoses, patients suffering from neurotic or organic mental disorders were most frequently and for the longest periods in somatic institutions.

Significant deviations between the means also became apparent in the study of somatic hospitalisations that had occurred due to injury or poisoning in connection with attempted suicide or were due, purely, to functional disorders. Due to psychological and psychiatric reasons, dependents and patients with neurotic disorders were treated most frequently and for the longest periods as inpatients in somatic institutions. It was noticeable that cases of affective psychosis, personality disorders, psychogenic reactions or heterogenic diagnoses were either rarely or never hospitalised for somatic treatment due to psychiatric reasons.

The analysis of the fraction of the hospitalisation time for psychiatric reasons produced only nearly significant differences ($p < 0.10$) where total somatic in-patient treatment was concerned. The fraction, approximately 3/5, was highest among dependents. The duration of hospitalisation required for patients with neurotic disorders due to psychiatric reasons was just under 1/4. For schizophrenics and cases diagnosed as affective psychosis and those without pathological findings, it ran to 1/5 of the total hospitalisation time in somatic institutions.

Discussion

The differences concerning in-patient treatment times and frequencies in psychiatric and somatic institutions were noted for patients classified according to different diagnostic groups during the follow-up period. Of all the diagnostic groups, schizophrenics were the most frequently and the longest in psychiatric treatment as in-patients, particularly where relative duration was concerned. The relative duration of psychiatric hospitalisation for schizophrenics was about 5 times longer than for cases with affective psychosis or with heterogenic diagnosis. It was about 10 times longer for the former than for patients suffering from a neurotic disorder or organic mental disorders. During a 15-year follow-up period, Williams and McGlashan [16], and McGlashan [1] also observed in a comparative study of different psychiatric diagnoses that schizophrenics and schizoaffective psychosis cases had significantly longer periods of hospitalisation compared with those suffering from an affective psychosis. Blumenthal et al. [17] observed a readmission rate 5 years after first hospitalisation which was higher by the schizophrenics than by patients with an affective psychosis, and a neurotic or psychosomatic disorder.

In contrast to this, Seva [4] observed during a 10-year follow-up period that the hospitalisation period was about 50% shorter in the case of schizophrenics in comparison to patients suffering from affective psychosis. However, only the in-patient treatment was registered at his clinic. Sund [3] found over a 10-year observation period that psychotics were more frequently hospitalised than patients with personality and neurotic disorders. His finding that patients with personality disorders were hospitalised in psychiatric clinics more frequently than patients with neurotic disorders cannot be confirmed in this study.

Our finding that schizophrenics were treated least frequently and for the shortest periods in somatic institutions could have psychopathological-like reasons. This would mean that there is a tendency to have such cases, when diagnosed as having a somatic disorder, admitted to psychiatric clinics as well. A further explanation could be that schizophrenics possibly pay less attention to physical disorders. Comparable findings from other authors [4, 16] confirm that patients suffering from an affective psychosis had considerably longer periods of somatic hospitalisation compared with schizophrenics.

The relatively long and frequent somatic hospitalisations of neurotic disorders can be partly explained by their psychiatric origin. This group of patients was hospitalised in somatic institutions longest and was one of the groups most frequently hospitalised for psychiatric reasons. The increased rate and duration of hospitalisation for cases of organic mental disorders in medical institutions is probably attributable to the increasing occurrence of simultaneous somatic phenomena brought on by old age.

Finally what is noticeable in the finding is that dependents were treated as in-patients for 3/5 of the total somatic hospitalisation period for psychiatric reasons. Furthermore, they were treated most frequently in somatic institutions for psychiatric reasons. An explanation for this could be the increased rate of attempted suicides by dependents, respectively alcoholics [18].

References

1 McGlashan Th: The Chestnut Lodge follow-up study: II. Long-term outcome of schizophrenia and the affective disorders. Arch Gen Psychiatry 1984;41:586–601.

2 Tsuang MT, Dempsey GM, Rauscher F: A study of 'atypical schizophrenia'. Comparison with schizophrenia and affective disorders by sex, age of admission, precipitant, outcome, and family history. Arch Gen Psychiatry 1976;33:1157–1160.

3 Sund A: The prognoses of psychiatric disorders in young Norwegian men. Br J Psychiatry 1973;122: 125–139.

4 Seva A: Psychiatric care contacts and follow-up (10 years) of 362 patients. Eur J Psychiatry 1987; 1:32–40.

5 Möller HJ, Schmid-Bode W, Cording-Tömmel C, Wittchen H, Zandig M: Schizophrenia versus affective/schizoaffective psychoses and prediction of poor outcome in schizophrenia. Acta Psychiatr Scand 1988;77:379–389.

6 Harding CM, Brooks GW, Ashikaga T, Strauss JS, Breier A: Vermont longitudinal study of persons with severe mental illness. I Methodology, study sample, and overall status 32 years later. Am J Psychiatry 1987;144:718–726.

7 Opjordsmoen S: Delusional disorders. I. Comparative long-term outcome. Acta Psychiatr Scand 1989;80:603–612.

8 Häfner H, Bickel H: Physical morbidity and mortality in psychiatric patients; in Öhmann R, Freeman HL, Holmkvist FA, Nielzen S (eds): Interaction between Mental and Physical Illness. Berlin, Springer, 1989, pp 29–47.

9 D'Elia G, von Knorring L, Perris C: Non-psychotic depressive disorders: A ten year follow-up. Acta Psychiatr Scand 1974;(suppl 255):173–186.

10 World Health Organisation: Mental disorders: Glossary and guide to their classification in accordance with the Ninth Revision of the International Classification of Diseases. Geneva, 1978.

11 Bleuler M: Die schizophrenen Geistesstörungen

im Lichte langjähriger Kranken- und Familiengeschichten. Stuttgart Thieme, 1972.
12 Kringlen E: Principles and methods in psychiatric follow-up studies; in Schimmelpenning GW (ed): Psychiatrische Verlaufsforschung. Methoden und Ergebnisse. Bern, Huber, 1980.
13 Ernst K: Neurotische und endogene Residualzustände. Arch Psychiat Nervenkr 1962;203:61–84.
14 Retterstøl N: Classification of functional psychoses with special reference to follow-up studies. Psychopathology 1986;19:5–15.
15 Berner P, Gabriel E, Kieffer W, Schanda H: Paranoid psychoses. New aspects of classification and prognosis coming from the Vienna research group. Psychopathology 1986;19:16–29.
16 Williams PV, McGlashan TH: Schizoaffective psychosis I. Comparative long-term outcome. Arch Gen Psychiatry 1987;44:130–137.
17 Blumenthal S, Bell V, Neumann NU, Schüttler R, Vogel R: Die Wiedereinweisung ersthospitalisierter psychiatrischer Patienten – Verlauf und prädiktive Einflüsse nach 5 Jahren. Psychiat Prax 1988;15:96–101.
18 Hawton K, Fagg J, McKeown SP: Alcoholism, alcohol and attempted suicide. Alcohol Alcoholism 1989;24:3–9.

PD Dr. Peter H. Vetter
Department of Psychiatry
University of Kiel
Niemannsweg 147
D-W-2300 Kiel 1 (FRG)

Psychopathology 1991;24:388–397

0254–4962/91/0246–0388$2.75/0

Erotomania – Erotic Self-Reference Psychosis in Old Maids

A Long-Term Follow-Up

Nils Retterstøl, Stein Opjordsmoen

University of Oslo, Gaustad Hospital, Gaustad, Oslo, Norway

Abstract. The concept of erotomania is discussed and the literature surveyed. The aim of the study is to present a long-term personal follow-up evaluation of cases with erotomania-like symptoms. In a material of 1,802 consecutively admitted patients, 6 (0.3%) presented symptoms suggestive of erotomania. They have been personally followed up 2 or 3 times by the authors over a period of 22–35 years. Our sample was characterized by avoidant and/or paranoid premorbid personality traits with difficulties in establishing relationships, and life-long social isolation. However, the overall clinical outcome was not hopeless. Neuroleptics may be of benefit, and our findings indicate the need for psychosocial treatment to increase the life quality in these patients.

Introduction

Erotomania is a syndrome where the hallmark is an elaborate, systematized delusion. The delusional belief is that one is passionately loved by another person, who usually uses surreptitious and covert means to signal his (her) devotion to the patient. Usually, but not exclusively, the patients are women from rather modest backgrounds. The 'lovers' are distinctly from higher social classes and financially superior (clergy, physicians, politicians, media figures). Usually, the patient will insist that the 'lover' has declared his love, and they describe in elaborate ways the glances, messages and secret communications that have taken place. Even if the patient first rejects the imaginary advances, she gradually accepts them and falls in obsessive love herself. The 'lover' is usually a married man who seems unavailable. The delusion of being loved usually lasts for years, and sometimes necessitates hospitalization of the patients or legal actions brought by the person who is the object of their affections.

Erotomania is also known as de Clérambault's syndrome, after the French psychiatrist who described 5 cases in 1921 [1]. However, Kretschmer [2] was the first to coin the same pathological state in 1918 as 'der erotische Beziehungswahn alter Mädchen' ('erotic self-reference delusion in old maids'). He described the 2 well-known cases of Helene Renner und Anna Feldweg, both presenting the typical symptoms. Kretschmer reexamined the 2 cases in 1926. The symptoms had gradually subsided, and the patients were unpsychotic, reverting to their normal selves as hypersensitive personalities.

From previous German literature Kretschmer found 2 reported cases: Wernicke's [3] school teacher from 1906 and Friedmann's [4] 40-year-old music teacher. The latter was married, it is true, but from an emotional point of view her situation was that of a spinster. Neither of these cases was quite typical of Kretschmer's new concept, however.

German psychiatry has elaborated more on the concept. Kehrer [5] in 1922 introduced 'Erotische Wahnbildungen sexuell unbefriedigter weiblicher Wesen'. He scrutinized the material from the Psychiatric Department, University of Breslau, and found althogether 6 cases which fitted into his concept. In all cases he found an interaction between mental and physical factors, personality structure and life situation.

Modern researchers usually overlook or are ignorant of the above pioneer studies. They are, however, aware that Kraepelin [6] subdivided delusions of grandeur into the delusion of being a great inventor, being descended from royalty, being a prophet or saint and erotomania (being loved in secret). Kraepelin gave a concise description: the patients are usually female and over 30 years old. He mentions that the syndrome progresses from the initial glance of the 'lover' through 'dreamy hallucinations' to obstacles and disappointments at the lack of progress of the affair. He also noticed about the course that the delusional content slowly diminishes, but the essential delusional content remains.

In spite of these pioneer publications from German quarters, erotomania has internationally been linked with French psychiatry and with the name of de Clérambault, because of his case description in his work from 1921: *Les Psychoses Passionnelles* (now only available through the 1942 edition of his *Œuvre Psychiatrique*) [1]. In the same year the English psychiatrist Bernard Hart introduced the term 'old maids' psychosis [quoted from 7].

The Present View of Erotomania or Delusional Loving and Its Course

Segal [8] has revisited the concept of erotomania. Even though he overlooks the studies of Kretschmer and Kehrer, his historical review is elaborate. As to the theories of etiology, he presents a range from Freud's notion of erotomania as a defence against homosexual wishes to Enoch and Trethowan's [7] theories on narcissism. Other viewpoints have been expressed by Hollender and Callahan [9], who note the physical unattractiveness of their patients, and Raskin and Sullivan [10], who emphasized that their 2 patients had recently lost their husbands, Seeman [11] separated a group with living lovers from a group with phantom lovers, and found the last group to have the most unfavorable course.

The literature is unresolved about the diagnosis of erotomania. It is also unclear as to the course. Kretschmer's [2] 2 cases recovered. De Clérambault [1] described a case where the delusion lasted for 37 years, while in Enoch and Trethowan's [7] 4 cases the delusion lasted several years, as was also the case in Hollender and Callahan's [9] study. However, there are also cases which are resolved after confrontation therapy [12], and there have been cases described where the symptoms have vanished and cases in which the patient gradually abandons the longstanding delusion only to fixate on a different object months or years later [13]. Recently Rudden et al. [14] and Gillett et al. [15] have pointed out that patients with erotomanic symptoms belong to different diagnostic groups, and that the course accordingly may differ.

Segal [8] has underlined that the new DSM-III-R category of delusional disorder, which is virtually identical to the original Kraepelian formulation of paranoia, properly includes erotomania as a separate subtype. He also points out, from his survey of the literature, that the delusions are usually persistent, but may diminish in intensity and shift to new objects. Finally, regarding the treatment, neuroleptics and enforced separation from the object are the best treatment options currently available.

Retterstøl [16] presented a material of 6 patients who had symptoms resembling Kretschmer's 'erotischer Beziehungswahn alter Mädchen'. After a follow-up period of 4–17 years, he found 5 of the patients to be nonpsychotic. All the cases could be diagnosed under the Scandinavian concept of reactive psychosis.

In the following, a new personal follow-up investigation of these patients will be presented, where the observation time period is prolonged to 22–35 years, giving the longest observation period which has been presented for this type of psychosis. Before the last follow-up the patients were diagnosed according to DSM-III-R [17] and ICD-9 [18] at index admission.

Material and Methods

The case records for all first-admission patients at the Psychiatric Department, University of Oslo, during the periods January 1, 1946 to March 20, 1948 (long-term group) and May 1, 1958 to March 23, 1961 (short-term group), were studied. With reference to the latter group, all patients were examined by Retterstøl in person at the time of hospitalization. The present investigation is part of a comprehensive examination and follow-up of all patients with paranoid and paranoic psychoses consecutively admitted to the Department during the two periods in question. Bipolars and confusional states were excluded. The material comprises all first admission patients who, during these two periods, presented a pathological picture resembling Kretschmer's 'sensitiver Beziehungswahn alter Mädchen' or Kehrer's 'erotischer Beziehungswahn sexuell unbefriedigter weiblicher Wesen'. The first follow-up examination took place in 1963–1964. All patients were seen in their homes by Retterstøl, who also had personal talks with the relatives in all cases. Readmission to psychiatric institutions for psychosis was furthermore checked against the Central Register for Psychoses, which records all psychotic patients admitted to psychiatric hospitals or departments in Norway [19]. The same author made a new personal follow-up of the patients in the short-term material 3 years later [20]. Later, all patients still alive were reinterviewed by Opjordsmoen [21, 22], so that the observation period was prolonged by 18 years (22–39 years observation period in all). Additional information from the Norwegian Central Register for Psychoses, hospital records, information from family doctors, and death certificates were scrutinized. The interviews at last follow-up were conducted using SADS-L [23] in the patients still alive. The overall psychosocial functioning was estimated using GAS [24]. GAS was also assessed retrospectively for Retterstøl's follow-up based on his clinical description [21]. The course in each case was estimated according to McGlashan [25] with longitudinal variables referring to the period of observation from index hospitalization to the last personal follow-up [21]. Interrater reliability for discharge diagnosis at index admission was estimated based on the same amount of information from the records for 2 raters [21].

The kappa value for DSM-III diagnoses was 0.79 and for ICD-9 diagnoses 0.64 [26]. Agreement regarding GAS ratings was measured using ICC (1.1) and

Table 1. Discharge diagnosis and global functioning at follow-up

Case	Discharge diagnosis		1st follow-up		Last follow-up	
	DSM-III-R	ICD-9	GAS score	observation years	GAS score	observation years
1	SFD	APR	75	17	deceased	22
2	DD	PS	67	16	?	35
3	S	PS	30	16	?	35
4	S	S	72	4	?	24
5	DD	PS	60	4	60	25
6	S	S	63	4	40	24

SFD: Schizophreniform disorder; DD: delusional disorder; S: schizophrenia; APR: acute paranoid reaction; PS: paranoid state.

with a value of 0.89 at Retterstøl's follow-up and 0.87 at last follow-up [21].

Of a total of 1,802 female patients consecutively admitted to the Department during the two periods, 6 (0.3%) presented symptoms suggestive of the above-mentioned condition, but not a single case could be classified definitely as a pure 'sensitiver Beziehungswhan alter Mädchen' or erotomania according to other classifications. The age during hospitalization ranged from 31 to 51 years (mean 40). According to the diagnostic classification used in the Department at the time of discharge, 4 had an uncertain diagnosis placed between schizophrenia or reactive psychosis, 1 had a diagnosis of reactive psychosis and 1 of schizophrenia.

Table 2. Course variables[1] throughout observation period

Case	Hospitalization	Employment	Social contact
1	3	3	3
2	4	2	0
3	4	?	0
4	4	?	?
5	1	1	0
6	4	2	1

[1] 4 Best, 0 worst.

Results

According to DSM-III and ICD-9 most patients had a discharge diagnosis of schizophrenia or delusional (paranoid) disorder (table 1). All patients were unmarried on admission and at the follow-ups. At the first follow-up 5 of the 6 patients were coded as nonpsychotic (table 1). Three of them had experienced no relapse after discharge, whereas 2 had suffered relapses from which they had recovered. In 1 case the psychosis had been chronic.

At third follow-up, after an interval ranging from 22 to 35 years, 1 patient was dead, 1 refused follow-up, 2 were untraceable and the follow-up diagnoses according to DSM-III-R in the remaining cases were delusional disorder and paranoid schizophrenia respectively.

Table 2 demonstrates some course variables and shows that the patients on average stayed most of the time outside hospital, went about their ordinary work during about half the observation period, and were rather socially isolated. Five of the patients stated that their nonmarried status had made them uncomfortable, as they felt different from other women.

The case histories will be briefly referred:

Case 1. Born in 1898, index admission for 3 months in 1946, followed up in 1963, died in 1968. Single, 47-year-old office clerk at admission. Two second-degree relatives had manic-depressive psychosis. Father a doctor (specialist). The home was described as good, harmonious, religious. Eldest of 3 siblings. Bright at school, matriculated for the university, studied economy at university level without examination. Secretary in office, very good at her work. No sexual experience. In winter prior to her admission she had moved to her sister who managed a hotel. Here she met an engineer, with whom she fell in love. Platonic relationship. The engineer was admitted to a mental hospital. She corresponded with him there, tried to help him by letter 'psychoanalytically'. One day she took a train to the countryside. When the train suddenly stopped because of a drunken man on the rails, she imagined it was 'her engineer'. She believed that God was behind the event, and that the engineer had wanted to deliver her a bouquet of flowers on the train to express his love for her. She was admitted as an emergency case, had marked disturbances of associations, improved on ECT, but relapsed and was readmitted 1 week after discharge, had to be transmitted to a mental hospital, where she stayed for 7 months. Later she was readmitted twice: in 1955 and 1962, both stays 3–4 months, mainly with depressive symptoms (major depressive disorder). Recovered. Fully employed, lived first with her mother, later with her sister. No sexual contacts, very religious, felt safe in Christianity. At follow-up unpsychotic. She said that her engineer was a married man, but had lived in a boarding-house in her town, while his family lived in another. She had not heard more from him, and was not occupied by this affair. Good insight. She died in 1968 of heart infarction, was unmarried, and, as far as we know, unpsychotic. Her premorbid personality was recorded as unremarkable.

Case 2. Born in 1905, index admission for 1 months in 1947, followed up in 1963 and 1983. Single, 41-year-old woman who lived in her parents' home, looking after them. No known hereditary tainting. Father a factory worker. Eldest of 3 siblings. Home condition described as good. Always meek and reserved, avoidant personality disorder according to DSM-III-R. Did well at school. Had been a cook at a hostel for some years, had remained at home for the last 13 years, cared for her parents. No sexual relationships. Three months prior to admission she complained that people talked about her. As a member of a choir, she was teased that there was something going on between her and the conductor of the choir. She got the idea that the said conductor was in love with her. People were preoccupied with her and the affair, and were after her, especially men. Not depressive – yet given ECT at the clinic. She recovered from the psychotic episode after 4 months. At the first follow-up she was unpsychotic, had been well all the time and looked after her parents until her father died before the follow-up. He had been insane during his last years. She lived in one of the flats in her parents' home, her sister in the other. She kept to herself and had little contact outside her family. She thought her illness in 1947 was due to overwork. She did not want to be reexamined in 1983, but wrote a letter. She then had angina pectoris, high blood pressure, and lived on an invalid pension. Her letter was very orderly and informative, indicating no psychopathology. She had not been admitted to psychiatric institutions during the observation period.

Case 3. Born in 1908, index admission for 2 months in 1947–1948, followed up in 1963. It was not possible to trace her in 1983. Single, 39-year-old teacher of domestic science. No known hereditary taintings. Youngest of 6 daughters. Father a teacher. She was spoiled by her father, and described herself as having an Oedipus complex. Relationship with mother not so good. Matriculated for the university after having failed 1 year before. Attended a domestic science school. Locum work at a number of schools, several jobs as housekeeper. Never settled down, repeatedly changed employment, continual conflicts with female colleagues. Touchy, sensitive, suspicious, easily hurt and annoyed. Painfully exact and tidy. Premorbid paranoid personality disorder with histrionic traits according to DSM-III-R. At the age of 20 engaged to be married, engagement broken off, nervous, though not psychotic. Casual sexual relationships with men. Hatred towards women. Had stolen a pair of stockings some years before, felt that people used this old theft against her, and that she was boycotted at the domestic science school. Felt she could not marry because her reputation had gone before her like fire in dry grass. Convinced that the headmaster of the school had fallen in love with her, and had definite plans about marrying her (no happenings could explain this delusion). Felt humiliated because she was not married, would not walk in the streets because of this humilitation. In the department she had the erotomanic delusion, felt persecuted by all women ('they were jealous'), had marked delusions of reference, was uncritical, and had slight to moderate loosening of associations and inappropriate affect. She ran away, and later insisted on being given a certificate stating that she had not been insane. Mentioned that she had followed the advice of some acquaintances that she should obtain more sexual experience, but she was incapable of exercising a critical judgement in this respect.

At follow-up after 16 years she was in regular employment as a charwoman. Extremely isolated in rented room, shy, timid, aggressive. She had had no contact with her family for the last 10 years. They had from time to time checked her address through the Salvation Army, but had not dared to visit her, as she then 'thought she was being persecuted and moved'. When her mother died, the family contacted her, but she did not answer. As far as her family knew, the employers were satisfied with her work, but she was on constant move.

In 1983 it was not possible to trace her, as she was constantly moving, but apparently took house cleaning jobs of very short duration. Based on the record at index admission this was considered a case at the border between schizophrenia and delusional disorder according to DSM-III-R. The erotomanic delusion faded, but she had long-lasting persecutory delusions, and probably has never recovered.

Case 4. Born in 1925, index admission for 3 months in 1959, followed up in 1963, denied follow-up in 1966, untraceable in 1983. Single, 34-year-old factory worker. Father and brother abused alcohol. Many difficulties in childhood home because of father's inebriety. Afraid of father, good relationship to mother. Number 4 of 10 siblings. Shy, inhibited, reserved from childhood. Total abstainer. Elementary school, did normally well, feelings of insufficiency because she had received no further education. Domestic service and factory work. Lonely, isolated. Lived in rooms in the capital. Paranoid and avoidant traits according to DSM-III-R. From the age of 19 she had gone steady with a boy, and had practically been engaged when her boyfriend suddenly left her and married another. Headache, restless after this event. Later she had a couple of casual sexual relations. After her broken engagement, she was very bothered by sexual thoughts and masturbated regularly. During the spring of 1958 she noticed that a work mate, 7 years her junior, affected her even when he was not in the same room. She felt he caressed her, and had erotic sensation in connection with this. During summer 1958 she kept company with this man for about a month, had coitus with him twice. After this she had no contact with him beyond casual chatter in the factory. From the summer of 1958 she felt exposed to him continually, either as caresses or patting on arms and legs. Felt his penis inside her all the time, as though they were having coitus. Experienced this so vividly that she got orgasms at work. During autumn 1958 she had lain on the floor of her room with spasms in her whole body because of the influence of this man, 'just like a wild coitus'. When she experienced the caresses, she concentrated on reciprocating them. 'He can make me do anything'. When admitted to the clinic, she was slightly depressed, reserved, incorrigible in her sexual delusions, delusions of being controlled and tactile hallucinations. Upon ECT and large doses of chlorpromazine the symptoms were reduced, but still present, so she decided to apply for work elsewhere, so as not to come under his influence again. At follow-up in 1963, after 4 years, she had been fully employed all the time. She moved from the factory after discharge, later worked as a deputy housewife, liked the jobs, lived in rooms. She would have liked to get married, but felt herself 'too critical'. Unpsychotic, thought her illness had been due to her unrequited love.

On contact in 1966 for a new follow-up, she asked not to be contacted, but sent a letter with the information that she was in full work as deputy housewife, and had a big flat of her own with which she was very satisfied. She was not traceable in 1983. However, she has not been admitted to psychiatric institutions again, and probably functions moving in her home-help jobs.

Case 5. Born in 1907, index admission for 14 days in 1959, followed up in 1963, 1967 and 1984. Single,

51-year-old woman, living at home, looking after her parents. No known hereditary tainting. Father smallholder, strict, difficult, domineering. She was afraid of him, better relationship with her mother. Eldest of 2 children, brother 7 years younger. Dominated by him in childhood. Disharmony in the home. She had always been difficult, sensitive, niggard, exaggeratedly clean, got what she wanted by persistent bothering. Paranoid and compulsive premorbid traits. Elementary school, housekeeping school, did well. Mostly stayed at home and cared for her parents, except for 10 months, when she was employed as a housemaid and cook. Serious quarrels with her father, mother had to act as a go-between. After her father's death 5 years prior to the patient's admission, she had become increasingly difficult. Domineered her mother, who had to submit to the patient's will. Tense relationship to brother. Very religious, actively engaged in mission work. No sexual contacts, not interested in men. Often ill during the latter years. 1954–1958: operation for ovarian cyst, varicose veins and abrasio. During her stay in hospital in 1958 she thought something was going to happen, felt tested in various ways. Everything that happened was a test. All this was because she was going to marry the local vicar. He was already married, therefore all these tests. She had to be careful. He had given her signs in the church, eye messages. The stay in the department was also a test. Afterwards she would see the plan for the marriage which the vicar was preparing. The symptomatology faded on chlorpromazine and supportive therapy, though she did not obtain insight. Discharged to her home. At the first follow-up, after 4 years, it turned out that she had managed well until her mother died in 1962. She had dominated her mother, refused to let her go to doctor.

After the death of her mother she felt persecuted by neighbors, admitted to psychiatric hospital the same year, stayed there 4 months without definite psychiatric symptoms. Discharged home. At first follow-up in 1963 no psychotic symptoms, but refused to speak about the vicar. Considered to behave adequately by those in her environment. Looked after herself in the parent home. The same appearance at follow-up in 1967, but she then stayed in a nursing home. At follow-up in 1984 in the nursing home where she had stayed since the sixties. Her brother did not want to have her at home, and she had been unable to care for herself. Still on a small chlorpromazine dose. Relatively good contact, listened to radio, read the Bible, behaved adequately. No insight in previous disorder, but without active psychotic symptoms. Unmarried. On invalid pension. Her doctor and nurse had the opinion that the patient wanted to stay at the nursing home because of the supporting and understanding milieu where she could avoid provocations and intense relationships. She was looked upon as 'strange', but not delusional.

Case 6. Born in 1929, index admission for 1½ months in 1959, followed up in 1963, 1967 and 1983. Single 29-year-old cook, considerable hereditary tainting: altogether 3 second-degree relatives psychotic, 2 schizophrenics and 1 delusional disorder, mother and sister nervous. Father farmer, had cleared the ground for cultivation himself, very strict. Poor relationship between the parents, much quarrelling. Eldest of 5 siblings. Elementary school, continuation school and 6 months' business school. Did well. Had mostly worked as a cook in hospitals and institutions. Always meek, quiet, unsure of herself, shy, afraid of new contacts. Avoidant premorbid traits according to DSM-III-R. A couple of sexual contacts from the age of 19 until she met a dairy apprentice when she was 24, and kept company with him. He broke off their friendship 4 years before her admission. She took this very much to heart. She never gave up the hope that he would come back. About Christmas time 1958 she saw from the newspapers that he had married. From January 1959 she began to hear this man calling her. She thought he was down in the basement of the hospital where she worked, and that he wanted her back. Someone had teased her about it. Voices informed her about his return. They suggested coitus, which she refused. Her friend was behind, wanted her back. During her stay in the department, she had feelings of strangeness, emptiness, had delusions of bein controlled, inappropriate affect, auditory and visual hallucinations. Treated with chlorpromazine with little effect. Considered as schizophrenic.

At follow-up in 1963 she was in full employment. The first months worked at home, later outside home. Got neuroleptics from the local doctor, considered as normal by her family. Nonpsychotic, considered her psychosis had been due to her frustration that her friend got married. At second follow-up (1967) housemaid in her home district, from time to time hallucinated, on neuroleptics. At third follow-up (1983) she lived at home with her father. Stayed 8 months in a mental hospital in 1973. From then on invalid pension, aftercare from hospital and neuroleptics for the last 10 years. Hallucinated from time to time. Much dependent on her father. Still unmarried.

Discussion

In only one of the patients in the present material was the premorbid personality recorded as unremarkable. A common feature for the other patients was a nonconfident personality structure, paranoid and/or avoidant, which had made it difficult to establish contact with other people, and which might be one of the reasons why they had stayed unmarried. Three of them had reportedly never had a love affair. All but 1 had led a lonely life, characterized by isolation and withdrawal to a sort of niche existence.

The 2 definitely schizophrenic patients (cases 4 and 6) were the youngest at outbreak of psychosis, which was associated with the breaking of a love affair in both. In cases 1, 2 and 5, the frustrating life situation of an unmarried daughter in middle age living at home appeared to have represented a heavy strain, and for case 3 the unmarried status seemed to have been especially humiliating.

In addition to cases 4 and 6, case 3 was also (with some doubt) classified as schizophrenic according to DSM-III-R, while 2 patients (cases 2 and 5) were diagnosed as suffering from delusional disorder, erotomanic type. Case 5 at index admission had a rather monosymptomatic psychosis, and recovered, but relapsed later with a psychosis of short duration. The second episode was also monosymptomatic, but the delusional theme had changed from erotomania to persecution. Case 2 had persecturoy delusions in addition to erotomania when psychotic. The remaining case (case 1) was diagnosed as suffering from schizophreniform disorder with good prognostic signs at discharge. Shortly thereafter she relapsed, and remained ill for more than 6 months, meeting the criteria of schizophrenia. However, there were 2 cases of bipolar disorder in her family, and she recovered after ECT. Later she had 2 psychotic episodes fulfilling the criteria of major depressive disorder.

According to our findings primary erotomania is an extremely rare conditon, as confirmed by others [15, 28]. Ellis and Mellsop [27], through their 5 cases and an extensive review of the literature, raise the question if the pure form or primary erotomania does exist. Munro [28] reported cases of monosymptomatic hypochondriacal psychosis, 'primary' delusional jealousy, and primary erotomania successfully treated with pimozide. He claims that they have similar appearance except for the delusional theme, and fit Kraepelin's description of paranoia. He agrees that those cases are rare. Most erotomanic cases reported in the literature have been secondary to another psychosis, most often schizophrenia or major affective disorder. According to the exclusion criteria in our study, bipolar patients were absent, which may explain why we did not find any case with erotomania secondary to affective disorder.

The first 3 cases in our sample were admitted before neuroleptics were available. Two of them were treated with ECT, while case 3 refused therapy. Case 4 with fantastic sexual delusions and hallucinations was treated with ECT and neuroleptics, while the remaining 2 cases were treated with neuroleptics alone. The long-term course of the disorder was episodic in 2 cases, chronic in another 2 cases, and uncertain, but probably chronic in the remaining cases. The erotomanic delusions lasted up to 1 year in 3 cases, also probably for a relatively short time in a 4th case, and the duration was uncertain for 2 cases. Overall clinical long-term outcome was favorable in 2 cases, relatively favorable in 1 case, poor in 1 case, and uncertain but probably very poor in 2 cases.

In conclusion, the present study confirms that erotomania is rare, especially the primary form. All but one of our patients had deviant premorbid personality traits with difficulties in establishing interpersonal relationships, and they remained socially isolated. However, the overall clinical outcome was not always so hopeless. Neuroleptics may have some effect [8, 28], we believe in the secondary form as well, but our findings indicate that in addition much emphasis should be put on social support for these patients.

References

1 De Clérambault, G.: Les psychoses passionnelles (1921); in Œuvre psychiatrique (Presses Universitaires de France, Paris 1942).
2 Kretschmer, E.: Der sensitive Beziehungswahn (Springer, Berlin 1918).
3 Wernicke, C.: Grundriss der Psychiatrie; 2nd ed. (Thieme, Leipzig 1906).
4 Friedmann, M.: Beiträge zur Lehre von der Paranoia. I. Über milde Paranoiaformen. Mschr. Psychiat. Neurol. *17:* 467–483 (1905).
5 Kehrer, F.: Erotische Wahnbildungen sexuell unbefriedigter weiblicher Wesen. Arch. Psychiat. Nerv Krankh. *65:* 315–385 (1922).
6 Kraepelin, E.: Psychiatrie. Ein Lehrbuch für Studierende und Ärzte. 8th ed. (Barth, Leipzig 1909–1915).
7 Enoch, M.D.; Trethowan, W.H.: Uncommon psychiatric syndromes (Year Book, Medical Publishers, Chicago 1979).
8 Segal, J.H.: Erotomania revisited: from Kraepelin to DSM-III. Am. J. Psychiat. *146:* 1261–1266 (1989).
9 Hollender, M.H.; Callahan, A.S.: Erotomania or de Clérambault's syndrome. Archs gen. Psychiat. *32:* 1574–1576 (1975).
10 Raskin, D.E.; Sullivan, K.E.: Erotomania. Am. J. Psychiat. *131:* 1033–1035 (1974).
11 Seeman, M.V.: Delusional loving. Archs gen. Psychiat. *35:* 1265–1267 (1974).
12 Rudden, M.; Gilmore, M.; Frances, A.: Erotomania: a separate entity. Am. J. Psychiat. *137:* 1262–1263 (1980).
13 Taylor, P.; Mahedra, B.; Gunn, J.: Erotomania in males. Psychol. Med. *13:* 645–650 (1983).
14 Rudden, M.; Sweeney, J.; Frances, A.: Diagnosis and clinical course of erotomanic and other delusional patients. Am. J. Psychiat. *147:* 625–629 (1990).
15 Gillett, T.; Eminson, S.R.; Hassanyeh, F.: Primary and secondary erotomania: clinical characteristics and follow-up. Acta psychiat. scand. *82:* 65–69 (1990).
16 Retterstøl, N.: Erotic self-reference psychosis in old maids. A personal follow-up investigation. Acta psychiat. scand. *43:* 347–359 (1967).
17 American Psychiatric Association: Diagnostic and statistical manual of mental disorders; 3rd ed., rev. (American Psychiatric Association, Washington 1987).
18 World Health Organization: Mental disorders: glossary and guide to their classification in accordance with the ninth revision of the International Classification of Diseases (WHO, Geneva 1978).
19 Retterstøl, N.: Paranoid and paranoiac psychoses (University Press, Oslo and Thomas, Springfield 1966).
20 Retterstøl, N.: Prognosis in paranoid psychoses (University Press, Oslo and Thomas, Springfield 1970).
21 Opjordsmoen, S.: Delusional disorders. I. Comparative long-term outcome. Acta psychiat. scand. *80:* 603–612 (1989).
22 Opjordsmoen, S.: Delusional disorders II. Predictor analysis of long-term outcome. Acta psychiat. scand. *80:* 613–619 (1989).
23 Endicott, J.; Spitzer, R.L.: A diagnostic interview. The schedule for affective disorders and schizophrenia. Archs gen. Psychiat. *35:* 837–844 (1978).

24 Endicott, J.; Spitzer, R.L.; Fleiss, J.L.; Cohen, J.: The Global Assessment Scale: a procedure for measuring overall severity of psychiatric disturbance. Archs gen. Psychiat. *33:* 766–771 (1976).
25 McGlashan, T.H.: The Chestnut Lodge follow-up study. II. Long-term outcome of schizophrenia and affective disorders. Archs gen. Psychiat. *41:* 586–601 (1984).
26 Opjordsmoen, S.: Long-term course and outcome in delusional disorder. Acta psychiat. scand. *78:* 576–586 (1988).
27 Ellis, P.; Mellsop, G.: De Clérambault's syndrome – a nosological entity. Br. J. Psychiat. *146:* 561 (1985).
28 Munro, A.; De Clérambault's syndrome – a nosological entity. Br. J. Psychiat. *146:* 561 (1985).

Nils Retterstøl and Stein Opjordsmoen
University of Oslo
Gaustad Hospital
PO Box 24, Gaustad
N-0320 Oslo 3 (Norway)

Psychopathology 1991;24:398–401

0254–4962/91/0246–0398$2.75/0

Obsessive-Compulsive Disorders in Benin: Five Case Reports

G. Bertschy, R.G. Ahyi

Service de Neuropsychiatrie (Directeur: Prof. *R.G. Ahyi*), CNHU, Cotonou, Bénin

Abstract. We report 5 cases of obsessive-compulsive disorders diagnosed among a sample of Beninese psychiatric outpatients. This type of report does not support the idea that this disorder is very rare in black Africa. Moreover, it appears that the clinical and epidemiological characteristics are not really different from those described in other continents.

Reports on obsessive-compulsive disorders (OCD) among black Africans are very rare. OCD are not [1] or hardly [2] mentioned in general reviews concerning mental health in black Africa. In studies dealing with diagnostics among patient populations, the diagnoses are imprecise and limited to neuroses or anxiety disorders as a whole [3–8]: if they are not, OCD does not appear among the specific diagnoses of neuroses or anxiety disorders [9]. However, two exceptions are worth reporting: (1) the high rate of obsession, as rated by the present-state examination, among the population of two Ugandan villages found by Orley and Wing [10] and (2) a recent report by Gureje et al. [11] on 2 cases of OCD among 1,914 Nigerian inpatients. Moreover, Rasmussen and Tsuang [12] in their sample of 44 American patients with OCD report the presence of 2 black people.

We report here 5 cases of OCD among 351 Beninese patients followed by one of us (G.B) during a 14-month period spent as a psychiatrist at the neuropsychiatric outpatient clinic of the National University Hospital of Cotonou, Benin.

Case Reports

Case 1

A 23-year-old male student had his first obsessive symptoms 2 years earlier, when he was suffering from a major depressive episode. He was afraid to pass people he knew on the street without seeing them. So he began to stare at anyone he passed. Soon he became worried about what people would think of him as he stared at them.

At the time of consultation, he was no longer depressed, and his obsessive-compulsive symptoms had changed. Having to share a book with the girl who sat right next to him in class, he began to worry about his ability to read the book at the same time as she did, but without staring at her. So he trained himself to look discretely to the side without staring at people every time he sat right next to them. This behaviour quickly became compulsive. Every time he would sit between other people to attend a lecture or a religious service, he could not help but look to the side. Whenever he tried to resist, he became very anxious and tense. But when he acted out his embarrassing behaviour, he ruminated about what other people would think. Finally, it was difficult for him to be attentive during lectures, and every time he could, he tried to find a seat at the end of the row in order to limit his embarrassment.

Obsessive-compulsive and avoidant premorbid personality traits could be noticed.

Case 2

A 25-year-old unemployed man had presented 6 and 2 years earlier two acute psychotic episodes with mixed affective features from which he had completely recovered.

When we saw him, he had no affective or schizophrenic symptoms. He complained that for a few months, almost every day, sometimes even twice a day, the following phenomenon occurred: he felt compelled to remember and to name all the friends and fellows he knew or had known. Such an operation took him 1–3 h. If he tried to resist, he felt a great discomfort.

It appeared that for several years he had minor rituals concerning folding of clothes or placing the doorknobs in what he considered to be their right angle. Furthermore, he had a marked obsessive-compulsive personality.

Case 3

A 34-year-old male civil servant had always been disgusted by dirt or excrements. He had even developed phobic behaviour concerning the excrements of his own young children. Since the beginning of adulthood he had minor rituals such as washing his hands after having touched a doorknob in a public place.

A few months earlier, visiting his father, he felt a great disgust, with nausea and even vomiting, at the sight and the smell of duck excrements in his father's yard. Since then, every time his mind was not busy, he could not help but remember the scene and to feel nauseous and vomit. Particularly propitious circumstances presented themselves while attending a meeting at work. Consequently, the patient developed a phobia-like anxiety for such situations. Every time he had to be in a meeting room, he tried to sit near the toilets or the exit for fear of sudden vomiting induced by such obsessive thoughts.

He had no previous or present depression. We could notice a premorbid obsessional personality.

Case 4

A 21-year-old male student who had suffered from a major depressive episode 6 years earlier. Since then, he has had intermittent minor depressive disorders.

Also at the age of 15 years he became disturbed by urges to smile at inappropriate times. At the same time he began daily ruminations concerning the adequateness of his behaviour and his religious convictions: any recent event could be the source of a kind of inner debate, lasting from 15 to 30 min and making him mentally exhausted at the end. Finally, clinical inquiry showed that he was also preoccupied with dirt and contamination. He refused to eat at the university restaurant because the forks were not always well cleaned. When he ate a piece of cake without carefully washing his hands, he would not eat the part which had been in contact with his hands; such a behaviour, particularly in the African context, always amazed his fellows. Furthermore, aside from being orderly and meticulous, he had no other features of obsessional personality.

Case 5

A 35-year-old male civil servant. His OCD had started at the beginning of adolescence with doubts concerning very basic mathematical rules or elementary knowledge in geography. However, these did not really affect his academic results.

After several years of spontaneous remission, the OCD reappeared when he started professional life. The symptoms consisted of checking rituals. Their intensity was moderate and their evolution intermittent. When we saw him, he was in charge of looking the doors and drawers of his ward at the end of the day. When he left, he was regularly invaded by doubts concerning such an action and had to come back to his ward to check it. He repeated this checking routine three of four times. The whole operation took him on average 20 extra minutes every day.

He also suffered from intermittent minor depressive disorders. There was a frequent but inconstant association between depressive and obsessive-compulsive perids. Apart from a certain meticulosity there were no clear obsessional features.

Discussion

These 5 cases represent 1.4% of a sample of patients attending an outpatient psychiatric clinic. Such a rate is similar to those seen in similar institutions in western countries [12].

The clinical aspect seems not to be different from that described in western [13, 14] or Indian [15] patients. The symptoms included obsessions concerning behaviour (cases 1 and 4), rituals of counting (case 2), urges to act out embarrassing behaviour (cases 1 and 4), obsessions of doubts and checking rituals (case 5), and obsession of dirt and contamination (cases 3 and 4). For the 3rd patient the association of neurovegetative manifestations (vomiting) with obsessional remembrance was somewhat more atypical, but the whole is clearly linked to dirt obsessions. All patients fulfilled the DSM III-R criteria for OCD [16], except case No. 5 whose daily symptoms did not last long enough.

The young age at the beginning of the illness, the frequent but not constant association with premorbid obsessional personality features, and the frequent comorbidity of affective disorders agree with western data [12, 13]. The lack of women in our sample cannot be further commented on because of the very low number of patients.

Perhaps we can quote the opinion of German [2] as a conclusion: 'When epidemiological studies of neurotic disorders in Africa are conducted with great care and precision there will emerge evidence to suggest that emotional and psychological patterns have a fundamental consistency irrespective of human race and pattern.'

References

1 Odejide AO, Oyewunmi LK, Ohaeri IU: Psychiatry in Africa: An overview. Am J Psychiatry 1989; 146:708–716.
2 German GA: Mental health in Africa. II. The nature of mental disorders in Africa today. Br J Psychiatry 1987;151:440–446.
3 Ben-Tovim DI: DSM III in Botswana: A field trial in a developing country. Am J Psychiatry 1985; 142:342–345.
4 Dhadphale M, Ellison RH, Griffin L: The frequency of psychiatric disorders among patients attending semi-urban and rural general out-patient clinics in Kenya. Br J Psychiatry 1983;142: 379–383.
5 Ebigbo PO, Ihezue UH: Uncertainty in the use of western diagnostic illness categories for labelling mental illness in Nigeria. Psychopathol Afr 1982; 18:59–74.
6 Johnson FYA: Mental disorder in JOS, Plateau State, Nigeria. History and admission statistics from 1974 to 1980. Psychopathol Afr 1983;19:69–82.
7 Onyeama WPJC, Onuora AN: A prospective study of 314 new patients referred to the psychiatric hospital at Enugu, Nigeria. Psychopathol Afr 1980;16:321–332.
8 Rwegellera GGC, Mambwe CC: Diagnostic classification of first ever admissions to Chainama Hills Hospital, Lusaka, Zambia. Br J Psychiatry 1977;130:573–580.
9 Cox JL: Psychiatric morbidity and pregnancy: A controlled study of 263 semi-rural Ugandan women. Br J Psychiatry 1979;134:401–405.
10 Orley J, Wing JK: Psychiatric disorders in two African villages. Arch Gen Psychiatry 1979;36: 513–520.
11 Gureje O, Osuntokun BO, Makanjuola JDA: Neuropsychiatric disorders in Nigerians: 1,914 consecutive new patients sen in 1 year. Afr J Med Sci 1989;18:203–209.
12 Rasmussen SA, Tsuang MG: The epidemiology of

obsessive-compulsive disorder. J Clin Psychiatry 1984;45:450–457.
13 Insel TR: Obsessive-compulsive disorder: The clinical picture; in Insel TE (ed): New Findings in Obsessive-Compulsive Disorder. Washington, American Psychiatric Press, 1984, pp 2–22.
14 Rasmussen SA, Tsuang MT: Clinical characteristics and family history in DSM III obsessive-compulsive disorder. Am J Psychiatry 1986;143:317–322.
15 Khanna S, Kaliaperumal VG, Channabasavanna SM: Clusters of obsessive-compulsive phenomena in obsessive-compulsive disorder. Br J Psychiatry 1990;156:51–54.
16 American Psychiatric Association: Task Force on Nomenclature and Statistics, DSM III-R. Washington, APA Press, 1985.

Dr Gilles Bertschy
Clinique de Psychiatrie et de
Psychologie Médicale
CHU St-Jacques
F–25030 Besançon Cedex (France)

Author Index

Vol. 24, 1991

Psychopathology

International Journal of Descriptive Psychopathology, Phenomenology and Clinical Diagnostics

Founded 1897 as 'Monatsschrift für Psychiatrie und Neurologie',
continued 1957–1967 as 'Psychiatria et Neurologia'
Founders: C. Wernicke and Th. Ziehen
Successors: K. Bonhoeffer (1912–1938), J. Klaesi (1939–1967), E. Grünthal (1953–1973), N. Petrilowitsch (1968–1970), Th. Spoerri (1971–1973)
continued 1968–1983 as 'Psychiatria Clinica'

KARGER

S. Karger · Medical and Scientific Publishers
Basel · München · Paris · London · New York · New Delhi · Bangkok · Singapore · Tokyo · Sydney

Drug Dosage

The authors and the publisher have exerted every effort to ensure that drug selection and dosage set forth in this text are in accord with current recommendations and practice at the time of publication. However, in view of ongoing research, changes in government regulations, and the constant flow of information relating to drug therapy and drug reactions, the reader is urged to check the package insert for each drug for any change in indications and dosage and for added warnings and precautions. This is particularly important when the recommended agent is a new and/or infrequently employed drug.

Printed in Switzerland on acid-free paper by
Thür AG Offsetdruck, Pratteln

Contents Vol. 24, 1991